A MIGHTY FORCE

Dr. Elizabeth Hayes and
Her War for Public Health

MARCIA BIEDERMAN

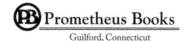

Prometheus Books

Guilford, Connecticut

⟨PB⟩ Prometheus Books

An imprint of The Rowman & Littlefield Publishing Group, Inc.
4501 Forbes Boulevard, Suite 200, Lanham, Maryland 20706
www.rowman.com

Distributed by NATIONAL BOOK NETWORK

British Library Cataloguing in Publication Information Available

Library of Congress Cataloging-in-Publication Data

Names: Biederman, Marcia, 1949– author.
Title: A mighty force : Dr. Elizabeth Hayes and her war for public health / Marcia Biederman.
Description: Lanham, MD : Prometheus, [2021] | Includes bibliographical references and index. | Summary: "A Mighty Force is the first book dedicated to Dr. Elizabeth O. Hayes's fight for public health on the American home front during World War II, for which she received national attention (and a victory under President Truman's Justice Department) for her protests against unsanitary conditions in the mining town of Force, Pennsylvania"—Provided by publisher.
Identifiers: LCCN 2021009209 (print) | LCCN 2021009210 (ebook) | ISBN 9781633887084 (cloth) | ISBN 9781633887091 (epub)
Subjects: LCSH: Hayes, Elizabeth, 1964– | Public health—Pennsylvania. | War—Health aspects. | War—Economic aspects. | World War II.
Classification: LCC RA807.P6 B54 2021 (print) | LCC RA807.P6 (ebook) | DDC 362.109748/65—dc23
LC record available at https://lccn.loc.gov/2021009209
LC ebook record available at https://lccn.loc.gov/2021009210

♾️™ The paper used in this publication meets the minimum requirements of American National Standard for Information Sciences—Permanence of Paper for Printed Library Materials, ANSI/NISO Z39.48-1992.

For Alan, my brother and oldest friend

CONTENTS

PROLOGUE

Three months after V-J Day and four months into a coal strike, Francis J. Erich was given an unpleasant letter to hand-deliver to a doctor. The letter came from the Shawmut Mining Company, which employed Erich, a large man, in a murky occupation. He described himself to census takers as a "special police agent," but he had no badge or license. He did have a gun, but there was nothing special about that.

So-called Special Agent Erich worked for Shawmut Mining in St. Marys, an attractive little city nestled in a north-central Pennsylvania valley. From there, Shawmut Mining's general manager oversaw its nearby mines, burrowed deep in the Allegheny Mountains. Yet the only addresses engraved on the letterhead were in the state of New York. The company was headquartered in bucolic Wellsville, just north of the Pennsylvania border. Its sales office was on the seventeenth floor of Manhattan's opulent art deco Graybar Building, high above Grand Central Terminal.

The first sheets of the company's letterhead gave the year of its founding, 1894, and a helpful descriptor: "Bituminous Coal." For lengthier correspondence, perhaps to keep the reader interested, a cartoon topped each subsequent page. Engraved into the header was a grinning groundhog reminiscent of Punxsutawney Phil, the end-of-winter forecaster of another Pennsylvania town, about an hour's drive south of St. Marys. But the rodents of the Shawmut Mining logo had a tougher job than their weatherman cousin. Standing upright in the illustration, with helmets on furry heads and picks perched on shoulders, they looked ready to dig all day and mighty pleased to do so.

Hence, every letter sent a message before a word was typed. The absent, wealthy men in control of the mine saw their workers as cartoonish, content with their lot, clothed but not quite human. Recently, however, the tables had turned. It was management that looked cartoonish. In words inked on newsprint and read worldwide, Shawmut executives were being portrayed as greedy pigs, wallowing in mud and releasing a stink strong enough to waft across oceans.

Today—November 13, 1945—Special Agent Erich would begin setting things to rights. He took the envelope on a twelve-mile drive to its recipient, Dr. Elizabeth O. Hayes, in a godforsaken coal town named Force. The letter gave her five days to clear out of her quarters. Until quitting in mid-July to enormous fanfare, Hayes had been Shawmut Mining's company doctor. Now she was their nemesis.

Three hundred and fifty men from Force had followed the doctor off the job. They refused to go into the mines without a doctor on hand, and Hayes was the only one for miles around. Hayes's tough talk about the filth of their coal town had catapulted her to media stardom. From Toronto to Manila, headline writers vied to write the most stomach-turning descriptions of Shawmut's "sewage-sodden" "toilet towns."

Editorial writers declared these hovels unfit for human habitation. The consensus spanned the political spectrum, including some papers that normally cared no more about miners than they did about groundhogs. But the spokeswoman for this cause was nothing like the stereotypical hillbillies of the popular "Li'l Abner" comic strip, a fixture of the same papers now championing Hayes. Though born and raised in the Pennsylvania hollows, Dr. Betty Hayes was a smartly dressed, wisecracking career woman out of a Jean Arthur or Rosalind Russell film.

Now, the mining company thought it had a way to get rid of her. Long after handing in her resignation, Hayes was still in Force, seeing patients in her company-owned house and going out on dozens of daily house calls. After negotiations with the miners resulted in assurances of their unified support, she agreed to stay put. As the only physician in a fifteen-mile radius, she could drive a hard bargain. The nearest hospital was in DuBois, eighteen miles to the southwest. An ambulance once sank in the mud of a mining-town road. In all its decades of collecting rents, Shawmut had never paved the streets. The only amenity introduced since the start of the century was electricity, added to homes when it came to the mines. The byways remained dark.

As one of Elizabeth Hayes's sisters, Catherine, remarked from her own medical office in Philadelphia, the area was "no place for a girl anyway. It has no future, no social life and has too much territory."[1] In that territory lived four thousand people, many of them pregnant, sick, ill-nourished, or fond of handling firearms. The miners among them faced daily risks of crushing, explosions, and drowning.

To thousands of others who read the papers, she was now the "Dr. Betty" of countless column inches. At thirty-three, she'd been christened the "girl-doctor." Just weeks after the Nazi surrender, she'd launched a new fight for democracy. In June, a suspected typhoid case had prompted Hayes to pay for private testing of the wells that provided Force with drinking water. Lab results showed that most wells were contaminated, a surprise to no one. The company had long done nothing to maintain the outhouses, and when hard rains fell, feces flowed down the streets and alleys.

With the company refusing to act and state health authorities sitting on their hands, the doctor and her allies went into battle. Hayes quit, demanding sanitation. The miners won back her services by walking out of the pits. The press called their goal the American standard of living. Shawmut Mining called it impossible.

Hence, Erich had drawn today's highly unusual work assignment. Company cops routinely delivered five-day warnings to families in coal towns. Even men injured in mining accidents might be ejected from housing if unable to work due to disability. It was something else, however, to hand this letter to a celebrity.

Astonished by her overnight fame, Hayes compared it to the craze wrought by the Dionne quintuplets' birth in the depths of the Great Depression. "We never dreamt that people would take such an interest in our local problems," Hayes told a journalist from the *Daily Worker*, the news organ of the Communist Party USA.[2] An editor hitchhiked to Force in the early morning hours, but with the Cold War already begun, he found the miners reluctant to talk.

Hayes, on the other hand, chatted briefly with the visiting communist; however, she declined to let him photograph her. The overnight sensation handled the media like a seasoned pro. Always quotable but often limiting herself to a few talking points, she kept her guard up with all but a few journalists. Still, virtually every outlet from the *New York Times* to the *Socialist Call* to *Newsweek* presented her case sympathetically. Some editorial writers and gossip columnists practically waxed worshipful.

After the Depression and the war, there was a general sense that Americans shouldn't live this way. An editorial in the *Philadelphia Record*, a big-circulation daily, declared, "The prescription of Dr. Hayes—'*Get good and mad—and start fighting*'—reminds us that many, many more Americans need to follow her example. There are a lot of Forces in this country."[3]

Anticipating today's cries of fake news, the affronted president of Shawmut Mining, John D. Dickson, characterized all these varying news outlets as the "yellow press." Dickson didn't sign the quit-premises letter to Hayes, leaving that to his general manager in St. Marys. In other places, such a letter might be just a first step toward eviction, with defenses available to the tenant. But in Elk County, even at the dawn of the Atomic Age, the mining company was both the landlord and the law.

On his drive to Force, Erich would have been treated to spectacular views. The coal camp was situated in Bennett's Valley, a thirty-mile sweep of Elk, Clearfield, and Cameron Counties with magnificent forest. The native elk were gone—hunted into extinction—but deer were plentiful, leaping through the laurel. The scene changed abruptly as Shawmut property loomed into sight. Foliage gave way to railroad tracks with a tipple, or loading structure, stretched over them. Then there was the "patch" with the miners' housing.

Centered in Force, the strike also involved two neighboring hamlets, Byrnedale and Hollywood. The men who worked Shawmut's two idled mines lived in one of these camps, as some called them, built at the dawn of the century. In 1904 a consultant advised Shawmut to avoid costs by selling lots to the miners, who could build their own houses. But mining companies saw the beauty of taking rents directly from paychecks. The houses, which cost about $500, were paid for many times over, and the workers were kept in thrall.

Architects called the style "vernacular." These houses were machines for living, now busted. Each had a sagging porch, a coal shed in the front yard, and an oozing outhouse in the back. Water came from wells, typically pumped by women and children in a daily backbreaking ritual.

It was nothing like Erich's leafy neighborhood in St. Marys, where his wife shopped at a grocery store just steps from their home. The only choice here when the roads were bad was the company store. Like other "rob shops," as they were called, the Shawmut Commercial Company recouped much of the miners' earnings, extending credit while disguising interest in its hiked-up prices. For spiritual needs, there was St. Joseph's Roman Catholic Church. Built by Shawmut to lure Polish and Italian workers, it was overseen by a cleric regarded by some as a company priest. Recreational offerings were limited, but anyone seeking a game of craps could usually find one under the church steps. For relief from the inevitable boredom, there was always the bar at the Force Hotel.

Like other coal camps, Force had its version of a silk-stocking district with lodging more suitable for the mine superintendent, priest, chief electrician, and other local elite. Erich's destination was known locally as the "big doc's house." Twice the size of the miners' homes, it boasted bay windows, a wide veranda, and a mansard-style gabled roof—but its chief distinction was indoor plumbing.

Dr. Betty Hayes had grown up in this house, a daughter of the previous company doctor, Leo Zeno Hayes. When her father first came to Force, it at least had a new coat of red paint. Built to last only until the coal was mined out, Force had the bad luck to exceed expectations. Shawmut's Proctor No. 1 and No. 2 mines continued to yield, but the weatherboard houses built for the workers settled and cracked, and human waste escaped the privy walls.

Three months before, Hayes had been rolling rugs, crating dishes, and filling attentive reporters' ears with her reasons for quitting. "I see no point in maintaining Well Baby Clinics if we are going to mix the babies' formulas with toilet water," she told one paper.[4] To another, she observed that kids playing in the backyards of Force sometimes made mud pies with human waste.

The miners and the media had convinced her to stay, but the rugs and dishes were gone anyway. By the time Erich arrived at the big doc's house, it was nearly barren. Once teeming with eight Hayes children, six bound for medical school and two for related professions, it now served only as a doctor's office. Hayes ate and slept at a miner's home, keeping only a few dresses here for days when she was too tired to budge.

Erich would have found it unlocked. It always was, even outside the office hours indicated on a little cardboard clock. Crime was rare in Force, as the miners had proudly told the press. Still, company cops were kept busy, materializing during housing disputes or when the occasional fight broke out. Known also for serving as the eyes and ears of management, some coal communities dubbed them "pussyfoots" or, more recently, "the Gestapo." Four months into a strike, people were anxious and hungry. In a place where no outsider's arrival went unnoticed, Erich was behind enemy lines.

Carrying 240 pounds on a six-foot-one frame, Shawmut's special agent could take care of himself. Before hiring on with Shawmut as a private cop, he'd served on a conventional police department in his nearby hometown, Kane. An avid hunter, like most people in these parts, he probably came armed. Firearms were commonplace in the households of Force, and for Erich, they were a personal passion.

Hayes's family members both hunted and healed. After a grisly hunting accident, Dr. Leo Hayes arrived quickly on the scene. He'd been close at hand, also stalking prey. In this forest-edged village, swarming with wildlife and ringing with gunshots, Leo was the woodsmen's medic. His house stood on the hill like a big red cross. Once, a man bitten on the leg by a rattlesnake had crawled five miles to its door.

Crawling in his own fashion, Special Agent Erich failed to find Dr. Betty Hayes at her office. He wasn't able to serve the notice until ten o'clock that night. Testifying about this first encounter in court, neither offered any details. It was soon eclipsed by a far more dramatic meeting between the two. On this day, a Tuesday, Erich may have waited near her lodgings until she drove back from a night of house calls. Or he may have tended to other business until knocking on the door of the house where she was staying. Either way, things probably happened fast, as they do in process-serving, with the server eager to escape before the recipient regains composure.

Did he check her identity, as process servers do, by first calling out her name? He'd been stalking her, sometimes from a distance, and she knew who he was. If it was their first brush at close range, Erich might have been checking the actual physician against the "pretty backwoods doctor" of the newspapers. They couldn't seem to print her name without mentioning that she was "young," "blonde," "slim," "attractive," or a combination thereof. So prevalent were these adjectives that one columnist, never having seen her, wrote that she "must be kind of a blond bombshell."[5]

But Erich submitted his envelope to a flesh-and-blood person of medium height and build. Measuring five feet, four inches, Hayes weighed between 110 and 125 pounds, depending on who asked and when. Photographed a decade earlier with a group of medical school classmates, all male, she is half a head shorter than most of them. One reporter, a man, termed her a "slip of a girl," while another called her "dainty." It all depended on the eye of the beholder; to another male journalist, she was "Nordic," "stalwart of build," and "all in all—a woman, the way you would say—all in all, a man."

Born on May 7, 1912, Hayes was two years older than the company cop, almost to the day. That slight age difference wouldn't have stopped Erich from sizing Hayes up against the pin-up the media had made of her. He'd married a woman four years his senior and bore no grudge against working women—unless, perhaps, they were married to him. Genevieve Erich left nursing to marry "F. J.," as the cop was known. The couple had no children, but she never resumed her career. A grocer intensely interested in *l'affaire Betty* wrote that the cop's wife came into his store daily, possibly out of sheer boredom.

As for Hayes, she played no part in the sexualization of her image. On one occasion, she covered her face with a clutch purse when flashbulbs popped. That only heightened her allure. Shortly after her June resignation she posed for an Associated Press photo. The picture, which ran for weeks in dozens of papers, is less than flattering. A crude penciled touch-up for overexposure broadened and flattened the base of her nose.

The result fell short of the bombshell mark. Still, it was a portrait of a white, groomed, middle-class woman, the type seen in postwar ads for electric ranges and refrigerators. Pent-up demand had consumers clamoring for those goods and the salary increases to pay for them. As the war ended, strikes broke out across the nation. Walkouts, sit-downs, and lockouts paralyzed Greyhound buses, halted New York City elevators, and silenced telephone wires from coast to coast.

To many, the least deserving of these discontents were the coal miners. The United Mine Workers of America had lost public sympathy by striking during wartime. But the Force miners were fighting for their health and that of their families. Moreover, no other labor story carried a photo like Hayes's portrait, fit for the women's pages or the society columns. One enterprising news outlet created a front-page comic strip, recounting the doctor's resignation in three panels. With big eyes and bouncy hair, Hayes's cartooned persona resembled other working women of the funny pages, like Dixie Dugan and Brenda Starr.

Now here was F. J. Erich stepping into the strip, the very caricature of a villain. He could call himself a company detective—one newspaper placed that descriptor between skeptical quotation marks—but such positions were prohibited by state law. At one time, the Coal and Iron Police, accountable only to their industrialist masters, had operated freely in Pennsylvania. But governors hadn't sanctioned these private cops since the early 1930s when their brutal murder of a miner sparked negative publicity.

If Erich was a relic of a shameful past, Hayes represented a bright future of clean drinking water, asphalt roads, and indoor plumbing. Most of her compatriots agreed that hardworking people and returning service members were entitled to these markers of the American way of life. That is, at least the white ones were. Company-owned mining towns had long been segregated, and all Force residents were white, according to the U.S. Census of 1940.

At the time Hayes took the letter from Erich, women were encountering pressure to relinquish their jobs to returning servicemen. Childcare centers subsidized by the government were being threatened with closure.

Women once recruited to the workforce by patriotic newsreels and patrolling neighborhood committees were now being shown to the door.

Betty Hayes was no exception. Physicians had always been rare in rural areas, but the war, with its huge demand for male physicians, had made her utterly indispensable. That had heightened her power while limiting her personal choices. With the men in white marching home again, Shawmut thought it had found a new opportunity. Her services were no longer needed, but her house was. Management was preparing to replace her with a man.

At times, Hayes's presence had been convenient for Shawmut, although she'd never been the company's first choice of physician. Now, however, they wanted her gone. New information about Shawmut's finances and Dickson's management of them had emerged in the Pittsburgh papers, embarrassing Dickson at his clubs in Manhattan and Wellsville.

These revelations might have caused panic, not just shame, in St. Marys, where Shawmut Mining's parent, the Pittsburg, Shawmut & Northern Railroad, was headquartered. (The missing "h" on the first word harked back to a failed attempt at spelling reform by the post office.) The railroad and its mining subsidiary employed large numbers of residents of that city. But for now, they were uninformed. Copies of certain Pittsburgh papers were burned, trashed, or otherwise disposed of before reaching the newsstands of St. Marys.

Undoubtedly, this had been done at Dickson's orders. Suave and restrained, the New York attorney left the dirty work—including the signing of eviction letters—to his Pennsylvania mine superintendent. However, letters written by Dickson show that Hayes incensed him. Initially viewing her as a seductive temptress, Dickson now saw her as the victim of a newsroom Svengali. Unable to believe she acted alone, he concluded that a "certain specific newspaper correspondent" had goaded her into publicly quitting to advance his own agenda. In any case, Dickson was determined to end it.[6]

It had taken generations to bring Dickson and Hayes to this point. Her antecedents were teachers and farmers who'd shifted to medicine when med schools were recruiting farm boys. Dickson owed his position to his father, a former lawyer for the coal-and-mining company, long in receivership, that his son now headed.

Counting from Tuesday, Hayes thought the deadline was the close of business on Saturday, a regular day of work in her six-day week. But the company executives, who didn't work weekends, expected her gone by morning. For more than half a century, the two sides had headed toward a confrontation. Now they weren't even speaking the same language.

1

THE INHERITANCE

The papers called Betty Hayes a "pretty heiress" because her father had left her his medical practice. Thrust it upon her, as it turned out. Five of her siblings had gone to medical school, but she was the only one still surviving and willing to take it on.

Her father's death was sudden. It happened during wartime, December 1942, and Betty couldn't make it home in time for the funeral. She was in Newfoundland, caring for poor fishing communities as a volunteer for the Grenfell Mission, the Doctors Without Borders of its day. The family cabled her with the sad news. Leo's battle against coal interests had ended when a lump of coal fell on his foot. The injury caused a streptococcus infection that spread to his brain and killed him.

Some heiress. Her father's $5,000 life insurance policy was supposed to pay double that amount for an accidental death. But death had occurred two months after the injury, and the insurance company refused to pay the additional amount. As the dispute dragged on, the company paid only $2,500, perhaps pressuring the family to drop the accident claim and settle.

Betty also took over the medical office in the big doc's house. In truth, the house belonged to Shawmut, but Dr. Leo Zeno Hayes had lived and worked in it for a quarter-century. The rented house was in Force's "silk-stocking district," as mining camps ironically called the area reserved for the physician, the priest, the mine superintendent, and other local elites. These residences enjoyed the luxury of indoor toilets and running water. They were typically built near the main road and the mine buildings, with which they shared a small water supply. The privileged few of Force got their water from mountain springs.

The village's other ninety houses were crammed together on hillsides. Practically identical, they looked like a heap of Monopoly houses—or would have, if game pieces included little outdoor latrines. Two dozen wells had been drilled to serve them, placed without regard to their proximity to the privies. Sewage seeped into the drinking water.

Now the entire festering mess was Betty's heirloom.

Her brother Vincent, a Philadelphia surgeon, stayed for a while, sharing the patient load and helping to battle the insurance company. His presence undoubtedly comforted his mother, with whom he was close. As her world caved in around her, Vincent was the only male left in the family and, many at that time might think, the natural successor to the father.

The unusual circumstances of their father's death raised questions about his deathbed wish. As the infection spread to his brain, he'd been rushed from Force to Philadelphia's Temple University Hospital, where Vincent was on the teaching staff. Efforts to save him failed. Realizing this, the dying physician expressed his last wish to his surgeon son. Betty was absent.

As told later by Betty and filtered through journalists, Leo Hayes had entrusted his daughter with the miners' care. In other versions, Leo's children were left to settle this matter among themselves. A magazine piece printed years later said that Leo had "managed to mumble" to Vincent, "I hope you children won't forget you were educated by the people of this valley. I hope one of you stays on until the people get permanent medical aid." Quite a mumble.[1]

The deathbed scene caught the attention of Woody Guthrie, the famous songwriter. In Guthrie's song, "The Dying Doctor," a heroic and sweet-smiling Betty shoulders the burden after the choice is left to her and her siblings. The lyrics describe Leo surrounded in his final hours by all eight of his children—even two sons who had died by then—and the gender count is switched from five daughters and three sons to the reverse. America's balladeer failed to imagine the Hayes family as it was: predominantly female, and jam-packed with doctors.

The reality was less a Victorian death scene than a game of hot potato. After a few months, Vincent returned to the medical office he shared with his other sister, Catherine, on 15th Street and Erie Avenue in Philadelphia. It was Catherine who described Betty's post as "no job for a girl." She was speaking from experience. Catherine had preceded Betty by one year at Temple University School of Medicine. Three Hayes siblings simultaneously studied there until Frank died before graduation in a vehicle collision as he drove home from an internship interview.

Catherine knew the terrain of Bennett's Valley, where she had helped save the life of a snakebite victim. The bitten man had crawled for hours toward Leo's door, only to discover that the doctor wasn't in. Catherine, then a medical student, grabbed her car keys and sped the man to the Du-Bois hospital. Recovering from the snakebite—and the wild ride to the emergency room—the man said he'd never again disparage "lady drivers."[2]

Catherine had assisted her father in Force after earning her medical degree, but she had no desire to take over his practice. Although unmarried and childless, she remained in Philadelphia after his death. Vincent, a father with a Temple faculty appointment and a wife from the Main Line, was even more rooted in the city. Helen, the eldest, had her own Philadelphia practice, not far from theirs, and taught obstetrics part time at Temple. Now a wife and mother, Helen had grown estranged from the family and was seldom seen at their gatherings.

Called to duty, Betty displayed her Temple Med sheepskin and her Pennsylvania medical license in the home medical office. They bore her full name—Elizabeth Omega Hayes. Her middle name, the final letter in the Greek alphabet, marked the close of a chapter in her parents' lives. "My grandparents decided that was it. They had enough kids," said Nancy Huffman, Hayes's niece.[3] There was no younger sibling to saddle with the job.

Betty's credentials had appeared in the Force practice before. The first time, they'd shared the walls with her father's documents. Four years earlier, after completing a year-long internship at a hospital in a suburb of Wilkes-Barre, Betty had spent about a year assisting Leo in his practice. Her first return—planned, rather than propelled by a sudden death—wasn't mentioned in news accounts or the Guthrie song. It wasn't a secret, but anyone in the know might have thought it diminished the sacrifice. If Betty had once returned of her own volition, was Force such a hellhole after all?

But Betty's previous return was part of a Hayes family tradition. Although the state didn't require residencies after a one-year internship, both Catherine and Betty spent time under Leo's tutelage before going it alone. Leo, too, had prepared for his first practice by shadowing an older brother, a one-time rural schoolmaster who had decided to go to medical school. A few months into her residency at Chez Hayes, Betty told local people of plans to open her own office in the Wilkes-Barre area, indicating that her partnership with Leo was always meant to be temporary.

Engaging with the community even then, Betty gave a talk on "social hygiene," as sex education was then known, to the female students of a high school in nearby Brockway. Her sister Aileen, married with children, was a school nurse there.

Back then, there was a third Dr. Hayes in the area. Gerald had opened a practice in Ridgway, the seat of Elk County. But first—following the

Hayes medical training system—he'd been a company doctor for Shawmut Mining, living with his own family in Elbon and close enough to Force for frequent consultations with Leo.

The warmth of family lightened Betty's prewar stint in Force. Gerald and Frank were alive then. Another sister, Leola, lived a few miles to the north in Emporium. The commotion of children filled the big doc's house every Sunday when Aileen's family visited after church. Nancy Huffman, a daughter of Aileen, remembers sledding down the hill behind her grandparents' house. In the summers, she and her siblings splashed in a tributary known locally by the ominous name of Sulphur Creek. "We knew there was a poor part of Force," said Huffman, whose visits were confined mainly to the narrow upscale slice of it. Unlike many children in Force, she didn't have to pump well water daily with an old wooden handle.

Even then, there were shadows at the doc's house. Frank's death left a first insurance nightmare like the one to come: the other motorist involved in the fatal crash sued for damages. And Gerald was already ill with kidney problems that surgery failed to alleviate.

In July 1938, Betty began seeing patients in Kingston, Pennsylvania, where she'd completed her internship. Just across the Susquehanna River from Wilkes-Barre, it was a three-hour drive from Force. Betty placed an announcement of her new practice in a local newspaper. It ran with her Temple Med School yearbook photo, a starkly lit portrait of her with braids tightly wound around her temples, mercilessly plucked eyebrows, and a forced grin.

She rented a floor of a two-story house for her residence and office. It was in the neighborhood of Nesbitt Memorial Hospital, where she had interned. Nesbitt had a policy of admitting one woman each year in its group of three interns.[4] Today, that policy might seem discriminatory, but it was remarkable for its time. In the 1930s, an average of 250 women graduated each year from American medical schools, but only 185 internships nationwide were open to females. In a dozen states, no hospitals accepted women interns. Yet many states required an internship for a medical license.[5]

Kingston boasted riverfront views. But Nesbitt's forward-thinking policy was probably the main attraction for Betty.

Betty's parents might even have encouraged her to stay in Kingston. It was one thing for Gerald to return home to Elk County from Philadelphia, where he had interned at Temple University Hospital. From his youth, he'd been an avid hunter, once costing Leo a hefty fine for illegally killing two deer in the first days of hunting season. He also had a family. For a young professional woman like Betty, the Wilkes-Barre area held more allure than Force, where the chief recreational activity was the craps game under the church steps.

Still, Betty's five years in Kingston didn't seem to hold her attention. As she set up her private practice on a quiet residential street, changes were roiling the world. As an intern, she joined a judging panel for a church-bazaar baby contest with scores of entrants. As the nation emerged from the depths of the Great Depression, silliness reigned. Betty also reunited with Penn State University classmates by joining the new Wilkes-Barre chapter of an alumnae group organized for female graduates of the coeducational institution.

Enrolled in a premed program, Betty had earned her bachelor's degree in science from Penn State in three years rather than the customary four. During that time, she'd formed a passionate relationship with a young lecturer named LeRoy Voris. Like Betty, he was from rural America, a preacher's son from Burgin, Kentucky. Neither would ever forget the other. It had the "energy of an early romance," said Larry Voris, a son of LeRoy, who'd heard his father recall it.[6]

Yet, the two separated. Although Betty was barely twenty when she left Penn State, and LeRoy just six years older, both were set on career paths. As powerful as their feelings for each other may have been, neither budged from those plans. Moving to Philadelphia, Betty began her medical studies at Temple, joining Catherine and Frank. Schooling or hiring six members of Betty's generation, Temple Med had evolved into a Hayes family tradition. She graduated in 1936.

LeRoy Voris remained at Penn State, teaching animal nutrition, operating a field station, and earning a Cornell doctorate. While Hayes was at Temple, LeRoy met another bright young woman. Eleanor Lathers had graduated Phi Beta Kappa from Syracuse University at eighteen. She'd taught there for a while before accepting a faculty appointment at Penn State, where she met LeRoy Voris. While Betty interned at Nesbitt, the couple had their first child.

Quite possibly, Betty was aware of this. Steak dinners with the local Penn State alumnae group may have kept her attuned to campus news while introducing her to other educated women. She also joined another group, the local affiliate of the National Federation of Business and Professional Women. Possibly, these memberships were an attempt to network and drum up patients for her new practice. But any business savvy Betty might have had was not evident in the launch of her practice.

She opened her doors in early July, an inauspicious time to attract new patients. Just a few weeks later, she closed up shop to take a vacation.

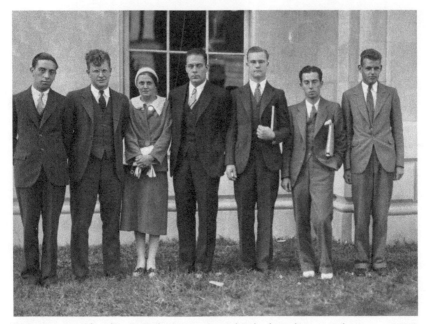

Betty Hayes with other Temple University School of Medicine students, ca. 1933.
Reproduced with permission from the Historical Society of Pennsylvania

Following the cues of medical schools and hospitals, many patients of the era preferred male doctors. Despite practicing in the shadow of Nesbitt, where hospital staff might have referred patients to her, she seemed off to a slow start. In late August, the number of physicians in Elk County rose sharply as Betty went west with an interesting companion.

The DuBois *Courier-Express* recorded the visit on a page filled with equally weighty news: "Dr. Elizabeth O. Hayes and Dr. Rudolph Marberg [*sic*], of Kingston, Pa., are spending a two weeks' vacation with Dr. Hayes's parents, Dr. and Mrs. Leo Z. Hayes, of Force, Pa., and with relatives and friends in DuBois."[7]

Like many newspapers of the day, the *Courier* regularly ran short items about visits, vacations, and other less-than-earthshaking events in the lives of its readership. This one was bound to have created a stir. With its freakish number of doctors, the Hayes family was always of interest. Now their young and attractive Betty had brought a man to meet her parents. *Courier* subscribers could put two and two together.

The reporter, on the other hand, couldn't spell the young man's name correctly. It was Rudolf Marburg, not Rudolph Marberg. As for placing him in Kingston, that had been his address for barely a year. He'd just completed his year of internship, a year behind Betty, arriving at Nesbitt soon after a ship brought him to New York from Antwerp. The ship's manifest described the twenty-five-year-old surgeon as a German national of "Hebrew" ethnicity.

The name misspelling suggests that someone other than the parties involved phoned in the item. As subsequent events revealed, at least one journalist based in DuBois found Dr. Betty Hayes interesting. The notice of Marburg's visit may have set tongues wagging, but there were no further developments. The two young doctors may have shared nothing more than a collegial friendship and a desire for a change of scene.

Even given the amenities at the big doc's house, Force was scarcely a vacation destination. Marburg had been raised in Augsburg, a picturesque Bavarian city, by his physician father and American-born mother. He earned his medical degree at the University of Freiburg, whose top administrator was the philosopher Martin Heidegger, a member of the Nazi party. After the anti-Semitic Nuremberg racial laws were enacted in 1936, banning Jews from professions including medicine, Marburg's widowed mother and his younger sister took a trip to New York, the mother's native city, perhaps mulling a permanent stay. A year after their return to Germany, Marburg immigrated on his own to the United States.

The Shawmut Mining coal towns were noxious eyesores, but their residents would leave Marburg alone. At any rate, the young doctor had few other places to go. His sister and mother had returned to New York for good, crowding with other relatives in an apartment. Given the circumstances, Manhattan in August wasn't an inviting prospect.

Meeting Betty's family and friends, on the other hand, might have been invigorating for all involved. In English learned in childhood from his mother, he could tell them about conditions in Germany, assuming that they asked. That was likely; Nazism and Hitler were subjects of great interest to Americans, many of them wary of war. Newspapers published in Pittsburgh regularly ran stories about Hitler's persecution of Jews.

Whatever they thought of his relationship with Betty, Marburg wouldn't have been the first Jew her parents had laid eyes on. Nearby DuBois had a synagogue and B'nai B'rith lodge. Moreover, Leo and Anna had spent several years in Philadelphia, home to many Jews. Leo's 1902 medical degree was from the Medico-Chirurgical College, or "Med-Chi," which had since merged with the medical school at the University of Pennsylvania. Admission to medical school, based mainly on the ability to pay, wasn't highly competitive in those days. Indeed, many entering students hadn't even attended high school. Exceptionally well qualified, Leo had finished teacher training. His farm background probably gave him an added advantage. Trawling small towns and rural areas for students—male only—Med-Chi recruited less vigorously in urban areas. Nonetheless, some Jewish- and Italian-sounding surnames crept into the rolls.

If Leo and Anna hadn't met Jews at the school, they might have encountered them elsewhere in Philadelphia. They had lived there as newlyweds, awaiting the birth of their first child, Helen, who returned to the city two decades later to break gender barriers. In 1925, Helen M. Hayes had been one of four women to graduate from the Temple University School of Medicine, which, though supposedly coeducational, seldom admitted female students.[8] Helen's yearbook commended the four for transferring to a "real medical school" from the Woman's Medical College of Pennsylvania.[9] Three-quarters of a century after Elizabeth Blackwell became the first American woman to earn a medical degree, derision and skepticism confronted those who came after her.

A Jew fleeing Hitler was the ideal houseguest for the barrier-breaking Hayes family. Leo had long sought ways to evade the mining company's authoritarian control of local agencies. To get roads and schools built, the company doctor had battled his own employer. Betty often spoke of Shawmut Mining as a feudal landlord.

But if she thought of the tall, blue-eyed Marburg as a life companion, it was not to be. After their return to Kingston, she continued with her practice and he with his studies. She visited the World's Fair in New York the next summer, two months before Germany—which didn't sponsor a fair pavilion—invaded Poland—which did. It was a rare foray outside Pennsylvania for Betty. This time, her companion was another young woman, the wife of a Wilkes-Barre used-car salesman.

Marburg eventually became a psychoanalyst. He moved to a suburb of Baltimore, where the leading newspaper would devote many column inches to the "pretty heiress" story. By then, however, Marburg had married.

Several months after introducing Marburg to her family, Betty lost another brother. After years of poor health, Gerald died at age thirty-three of hepatitis, leaving behind a wife and three daughters. There was no autopsy. Ironically, Gerald had been elected to a second four-year term as Elk County coroner shortly before his death. He was so ill at that point that he could barely run his medical practice, never mind campaign. But he'd once cared for mining families, and the name Hayes got votes. That was the valuable part of Betty's legacy, and she later would use this to her advantage.

It is unknown whether her relationship with a German Jewish refugee had anything to do with it, but Betty was passionately committed to the Allied cause. When the United States entered the war, women physicians were barred from enlisting as medical officers. Still, the draft changed everything. Unable to fill their seats with men, medical schools admitted record numbers of women. For those already licensed, like the youngest Dr. Hayes, there were new opportunities.

Her practice survived its rough start. She was still seeing patients at her Kingston apartment in May 1942 when a staff job suddenly became available at the Kirby Memorial Health Center in Wilkes-Barre. Recently built by a local philanthropist, Kirby was an architectural wonder of tile, bronze, and oak. Housed within this Spanish Mission–style structure was the state tuberculosis clinic, which was about to lose Dr. Donald C. Smith. Smith was due to report at the U.S. Army's Camp Kilmer in New Jersey.

Like Betty, Smith was not the only doctor in his family. A brother practiced in the home of their widowed mother, a mile from Betty's office, with Nesbitt Hospital the midpoint between the two. Whether seeking advancement or just eager for a change, Betty succeeded Smith soon after he went on active duty.

But the new position somehow failed to satisfy her. With five years of practice under her belt, she started at the state lab as an assistant clinician, although she would later say that she'd done surgical experimentation. Hired as Smith's replacement, she might not have been given his job title. Given Smith's army career—a major, he was chief of surgery on a hospital ship—it's unlikely that civilian life had made him a lowly subordinate.

Whatever previous form it had taken, Betty Hayes's job was an assistantship. Four months into it, she quit. Like many socialites and Ivy Leaguers of her era, Hayes went off to the Grenfell Mission in northern Newfoundland. Although founded by a British doctor, Wilfred Grenfell, the organization had evolved into a favorite American philanthropic cause. Its hospitals, schools, and daycare centers relied on support from a dozen fundraising chapters in the United States. Even after war dominated the world's attention, New York debutantes still flocked to Grenfell sites every summer to hoe gardens, can fruit, and sell used clothing.

If Betty's abrupt departure created inconvenience—as it almost certainly did in wartime—the local newspaper gave no hint of that in its coverage. The Grenfell Mission was associated with altruism. With clashes between the Red Army and the Nazis dominating its front page, the *Wilkes-Barre Record* offered this novelty in its suburban news section:

> Forsaking the comforts of a Kirby Health Center office, Dr. Elizabeth
> O. Hayes . . . has decided to pursue her chosen work, tuberculosis re-
> search, in Newfoundland, and will leave here soon. Dr. Hayes will go to
> the famed Grenfell Foundation at the northern tip of Newfoundland in
> the village of St. Anthony, just across from Labrador. In her new clinic,
> whenever she travels, it will be by means of dog team and sled, clothed
> in a parka of heavy fur.[10]

A mention of dogsleds never failed to fascinate the American public,
which lapped up news about the Harvard men and Vassar women who
were scrubbing floors and painting walls at the Grenfell's hospitals, orphanages, and schools. A stint of menial work at its Newfoundland facilities
was thought to be character-building for privileged American youth, who
volunteered mostly in the summer. Still known as a mission, the nonde-
nominational project had never been chiefly religious, but it promoted
good works.

The smaller number of volunteers who braved the brutal winters
described the harsh conditions while expressing a quasi-mystical desire to
return. Their remarkably similar stories, undoubtedly shaped by the Grenfell's public-relations machine, drew donations of cash and labor. Yet it's
unlikely that Hayes forsook her state job for a soul-purifying adventure. If
she had wanted to test her mettle in a remote, inhospitable landscape, she
could have gone home to Force.

It's equally unlikely that she expected her duties in Newfoundland to
be confined to research. Tuberculosis was, indeed, a scourge in that part
of the world, and the St. Anthony hospital—opened in 1927 with forty
beds—had since added a tuberculosis annex. Always run lean, it had a
medical director, one or two physicians, a handful of nurses, and a dentist
when possible. Hayes was sure to see TB cases, but did not tend to them
exclusively. She may have concocted the research story to explain her sudden departure from her Pennsylvania assistantship. It wouldn't be the last
time she felt pressured to stick to an unwanted job.

The Grenfell Mission offered an opportunity to burnish her credentials. Despite their remoteness, the main hospital in St. Anthony and one
down the coast at Twillingate were highly regarded. Graduates of elite British and American schools staffed the mission's hospitals, satellite, and nursing stations. Built to serve the poor, the main hospital also lured wealthy
patients from Newfoundland's capital, St. John's, six hundred miles away.
Given a stash of radium by a Pittsburgh women's club, the main Grenfell
hospital was the only site on the island offering radiation therapy.

No one went to the Grenfell for the money. The mission's staff famously worked for little or nothing. Indeed, the summer volunteers covered their own expenses, including travel. But at a time when internship and residency opportunities for women were severely limited, it was Betty's chance to join the staff of a highly accredited hospital.

The job took her from quiet, suburban Kingston to a ringside seat on the Battle of the Atlantic. Even before entering the war, the United States had leased three air bases in Newfoundland and stationed tens of thousands of troops on them. With British attention drawn elsewhere, the United States and Canada were tasked with defending the island, which was then a British dominion. Bombers flew overhead while German U-boats threatened Allied supply vessels bound for Great Britain and the Soviet Union. As Newfoundland became one of the most highly militarized zones in North America, the Grenfell Mission plunged Betty into the thick of things.

Peacetime likely wouldn't have offered this opportunity. Most physicians at the St. Anthony hospital were male, both before and during the war. In 1941, a female ophthalmologist had joined them, but just for the summer. Since then, the draft had sapped America's store of young medical men, already in short supply in Canada and Great Britain. Hence, the hospital position fell to Hayes. She escaped a posting to one of the mission's "cottage hospitals," four-room affairs in the mission's farthest reaches.

The Grenfell Mission had yet to enter the age of aviation. The aircraft crowding the Newfoundland skies were mostly reserved for defense. But the Grenfell was well equipped with ice boats, as well as its fabled dog teams. Grit and determination helped it deliver medical services to fifty thousand fishing families scattered along three hundred miles of coast. Its hospital boats kept schools and orphanages fueled and supplied to near prewar levels. In Pennsylvania, Leo Hayes had to struggle for years to get one road built. There couldn't have been a starker contrast between the Grenfell Mission's commitment and Shawmut Mining's indifference.

Leo's battles weren't over, but his part in them had ended. Betty received a cable with the news of his death. The newspapers said Betty took the first flight south, but that probably was no simple matter. It was December, not the season for the steamers that ferried passengers between St. Anthony and the airport in St. John's. In the winter, Grenfell workers had to await mail steamers for long journeys down the coast. Then came the trip to Force, hours from any major air terminal.

A large swath of Pennsylvania coal country was mourning Leo. He had tended mining families for forty years, picking up some Polish and Italian, while also fighting to fill their greater needs. Shawmut had transferred him for several years to Jefferson County, where Betty was born in the mining camp of Conifer. There, her father had worked tirelessly to build a sorely needed hospital. Just weeks before Leo's death, Brookville Hospital had printed a love letter to him in the local paper. Long after leaving the area, he still sent generous checks.

The doctor was buried in St. Leo's Cemetery in Ridgway. It was done by the time Betty arrived, tired and confused. Three days later came a letter that shook her awake. It informed her that the mining company had its own ideas about her father's legacy. "Do not plan to stay," began the letter, which was not about real estate. Eagerly accepting rent from anyone able to pay, Shawmut transferred Leo's lease to his widow. But it didn't want their daughter as the company physician.

News of Betty Hayes's plans had probably percolated from Force to the corporate offices. Next to the doc's house lived David Bell, Sr., the mine superintendent. Once friendly, the two families had hunted together. That was lucky for the Bells; Betty's sister Aileen was with the neighbors when Mrs. Bell accidentally shot her younger son, shattering his leg. Aileen, a nurse, administered first aid until Leo emerged from the bushes.

The leg had been amputated, and the boy was fitted with a prosthetic. Now an adult, David Bell, Jr., had a managerial job with Shawmut Mining. Despite the debt owed his neighbors, the senior Bell was firmly in the anti-Hayes camp.

Shawmut's general manager, Frank Lambert, and Dave Bell were loyal company men, while Leo Hayes had never truly been a company doctor. Coal-town physicians usually acted at their employers' bidding. They were known for minimizing reports of work-related injuries and for ordering sick miners back to work. Leo instead had opposed management to help build a school, a hospital, and a road. Shawmut had no interest in the future of the towns it had slapped up four decades ago. As is, they were serving their purpose.

For the company heads, Leo's sudden death was a boon. They had found a new occupant, presumably one who'd be loyal to them, for the big house on the hill. However, as Hayes learned from her own news sources, the would-be usurper was not a medical doctor. Shawmut planned to thwart her father's wishes by replacing him with an osteopath. With one-third of the nation's physicians in the armed services, this probably came as no surprise. Men with conventional medical degrees had been pressured into enlisting, even if draft-exempt due to age or other reasons. But osteopaths, like female MDs, couldn't join the military as medical officers. If drafted or voluntarily enlisted, they started with basic training, like other GIs.

At the time, the training of medical doctors and osteopaths varied more than it does today. For that reason and others, there was a movement to exclude osteopaths from membership in the American Medical Association. Hayes, who belonged to the AMA, didn't seem to think much of osteopaths, but others in the association thought differently, or perhaps they didn't wish to shed dues-paying members. Whatever the reason, the movement to eject osteopaths failed and they remained part of the AMA, heavily influential in setting professional training standards.

The government of Pennsylvania, home to several schools of osteopathy, didn't share Betty's contempt either. The state allowed osteopaths a wide scope of practice provided they passed an exam. Here was a catch that Hayes would seize upon. Shawmut Mining's candidate lacked a Pennsylvania license and had no chance of obtaining one quickly. The state qualifying test was administered only a few times a year.

Management's sneak attack backfired. Betty Hayes had been a reluctant heiress, but this move turned her into a militant one. Clearly, the company had grabbed the first job candidate willing to do its bidding. With Leo not yet cold in his grave, there'd been no time to check this person's background or contact references. Anticipating an outcome like this, the father had bound his children to a promise.

Betty took the matter directly to the miners. She contended that the miners, not the company, employed the company physician. Because the doctor was paid mainly through deductions from their paychecks, the choice should be theirs. Her father had apparently agreed with her. On the 1940 census, nearly all Force residents named coal mines as their business or industry, apart from the few employed by a store, church, factory, or school; however, Leo said he was in "private practice," departing from his answer a decade earlier when he said he worked for a "mining town."

Shawmut's small monthly salary didn't make him their creature. Lately, the company hadn't even bothered to pay it. When Leo died, Shawmut owed him $4,500, more than a year's salary, which it never paid his estate. Without the miners' paycheck deductions—$1.50 for married men and seventy-five cents for single ones—he wouldn't have had a dependable source of income.

Leo's reasons for describing himself as a private practitioner to a census taker died with him. Betty, on the other hand, made the same argument publicly, with immediate political consequences. Those who paid, she maintained, had the right to choose their practitioner.

The miners scheduled a meeting that united various factions in common cause. All Shawmut miners were members of the United Mine

Workers of America, hired according to union rules. Their union president was the bushy-browed, fiery John L. Lewis, described by one columnist as a "thespian" and "tragedian." After working to re-elect Franklin D. Roosevelt in 1936, Lewis had battled with the president over labor matters. Roosevelt won a third term in 1940 as Lewis threw his support to Republican challenger Wendell Willkie. Despised in certain circles on both the political left and right, Lewis was not universally admired here, either. As frequent wildcat strikes attested, no leader's word was law in the central Pennsylvania coalfields.

Skeptical of the union's top officials, yet firmly committed to unionism, 275 Shawmut Mining employees—three-quarters of the workforce—assembled to choose their doctor. Management, relying on its own notions as much as its hired snoop, didn't consider them indivisible. Their various religions, ethnicities, and ages offered potential points for the driving of wedges. Catholics gathered with Methodists. Middle-aged immigrants from Poland and Italy sat with American-born youths. They didn't necessarily work together. Residents of Force and Byrnedale mined Shawmut's Proctor No. 1 mine, while those of Hollywood—bearing no resemblance to its glamorous namesake—toiled in Proctor No. 2.

The houses hastily erected in the three hamlets were nearly identical, and their occupants faced the same problems of neglect and poor sanitation. But they were organized into different locals of the UMWA. Anthony Coccimiglio was president of both Local 97 of Force and Local 851 of neighboring Byrnedale. Born in Italy but raised locally, Tony was an amateur bandleader with a theatrical flair. The Hollywood miners belonged to Local 6397, led by John E. "Ted" Challingsworth, an immigrant from England still mining in his sixties.

Although separated by just a few miles, the villages had separate social orbits. Families of one hamlet were often linked to adjacent ones by marriage or blood. At summertime picnics, teams from Hollywood and Force competed on the baseball field. By all appearances, this was simply a good-natured rivalry, but underneath lurked fissures that could easily widen. The three communities also were in varying states of need. Force, named for frontiersman Jack Force, was in critical shape. Hollywood, although needy, was better off, and Byrnedale was somewhere in the middle.

On this day, however, the rivals put their differences aside. Employed in one of the world's most hazardous occupations and concerned for their families, they wanted the physician issue settled. The leaders agreed with Hayes that the physician should serve at the miners' pleasure. As it happened, Hayes's views on their right to choose matched those of the national miners' union, which hoped to rid itself of company doctors and establish a healthcare program granting workers the right to choose their own doctor. So far, though, Lewis's efforts in that direction had failed. There was nothing in the contract giving miners a voice in the choice of their physician, just as there was nothing to stop management from housing families in fetid hovels.

As the miners raised their hands—all for Betty Hayes and none for the osteopath—history was made. The coal miners of Bennett's Valley had taken their first steps toward a union-run medical plan. The day would come when the UMWA pointed to them as a model. For now, they were invisible, just a ripple in the sea of union members who occasionally penned letters to the famous John L. Lewis, receiving formulaic replies beginning, "Dear sir and brother," from one of his hand-picked district presidents.

The meeting probably took place at St. Joseph's Church or in its church hall, where a photo taken later shows Hayes addressing miners in a Sunday school classroom. The union hall wasn't available. The miners had rented their meeting place to an independent grocer, ending the company store's monopoly. Families deep in arrears were still forced to patronize Shawmut's "rob shop," but even there, competition and wartime regulations had tempered the usual extortionary prices.

Hayes, however, was stuck in place. Her victory left her where she'd started. She was living with her mother in her hometown. Three years earlier the World's Fair had shown her the World of Tomorrow, which didn't warn of fascism and a global war. Instead, it was a consumers' paradise as imagined by General Electric and Westinghouse, full of cutting-edge innovations like dishwashers and television. All that stood in the way was socialism, according to a promotional film about a fictitious family, the Middletons. The parents thrill to the exhibits while their daughter's fiancé calls them capitalist trash. In the end, the daughter ditches this leftist for a hometown boy, and fireworks explode.

There were no fireworks as the meeting of the miners broke up. After the church hall closed, the only light came from the stars and the small house windows across the highway. The roads up the hills were icy and unpaved. Anyone injured late at night would need to rouse Hayes with a knock. Phone service shut off at 9:30 p.m. and didn't resume until 7:00 a.m.

Now officially an heiress, Hayes had also inherited her father's car. Although the church was within easy walking distance of her home, she probably drove to the meeting. Women who pumped water in Force wore sensible clothes, long checkered jackets over skirts and boots, practical for lugging water buckets and avoiding hunters' gunfire. Hayes was partial to ruffled blouses, appliqued dresses, puckered sleeves, and veiled hats. These choices were typical of 1940s career wear, but they also expressed her taste and possibly a little vanity. The papers got some things right. "She was a pretty girl," one of several in her family, her niece Nancy said.

One particular ensemble would spark a need for further meetings. Hayes wore it as she emerged from her car to attend to a woman who'd gone into labor. Slipping and falling on a street that Shawmut refused to pave, Hayes rose with excrement all over her dress, and had to deliver the baby in that condition.

As the war went on, this story would reach the national desks of newsrooms, where it would resonate with a new wave of journalists. They were women, called in from the sidelines. New horizons had opened for them, at least for the duration of the war.

But not for Hayes. Now that she had secured her job against the company's wishes, Shawmut Mining intended to shackle her to it.

2

NO ESCAPE

The next challenge came from some of the same miners who'd voted to keep Betty Hayes as their doctor. They were summoning her to their bedsides after dark.

She would drive the treacherous roads only to find that the man had faked his symptoms. Hayes stuck with her job despite these multiple instances of sexual harassment—or sexual assault if, as is entirely possible, they involved physical examination. The perpetrators and the world at large viewed them as pranks of the boys-will-be-boys variety. "A few young practical jokers thought it was a lot of fun chasing an attractive girl around," was a typical summary of these outrages, which, aside from harming Hayes, made her unavailable for real emergencies.

Hayes was angry, as her harassers undoubtedly anticipated, perhaps also expecting her silence. That was not to be. She asked the union leaders to convene a meeting, where she announced her intention to charge five dollars, "collectible on the spot," for any such future incidents. Collecting that amount would have been difficult. It was more than six times the amount that Shawmut deducted from paychecks monthly for a single man's medical coverage. The leaders backed her up with their own threat, one that literally had teeth.

After Hayes spoke, according to a magazine writer, "Big Bill Agosti lumbered to his feet. If it ever happens again,' he said, '*my* fee is a busted jaw for the guy—also collectible on the spot.' It never happened again."[1]

Thus, Hayes made her conditions clear. As a physician and a woman weighing "112 pounds wringing wet," as the same writer put it, she couldn't threaten violence. Still, in calling the meeting, she must have known that the unionists would. With her father dead and her sole

17

surviving brother back in Philadelphia, she needed male protection to carry out her duties as a physician.

Because she'd been absent from Force for years, her young harassers might have mistaken her for an outsider, wearing kid gloves and flowered fascinators in a sea of flannel. "Big Bill," as the magazine described William Agosti, had known Hayes and her family for years. Of only medium height but husky build, Bill was so influential in Local 97 that one newspaper misidentified him, instead of Tony Coccimiglio, as its president. Anyone picking a quarrel with Agosti risked the wrath of many. Two of his brothers had married sisters, and all had parents and other relatives in the area.

Although unrelated to miners, the Hayes family was enmeshed in these relationships. Aileen and her husband, Ross Ferraro, had formed what would be a lifelong friendship with Henry and Martha Agosti. That friendship would eventually keep Hayes housed, nourished, and able to receive patients when those essential tasks became a challenge.

For now, there was her mother. Saddened by the sudden loss of her husband after the premature deaths of two sons, Anna by now was in her late sixties. For now, she could cook and clean for Betty as she had for Leo, but the situation wasn't sustainable. A year after the miners voted to keep Betty with them, the family helped Anna plan her departure. She filed for a permit to build a house near Aileen and her family in Brockway. The grandchildren would distract her from her grief.

Between deed transfers and weather delays, it was more than a year before Anna could move into her new house. In the meantime, she kept house for Betty, but Anna's life with her youngest daughter couldn't have been very companionable. As Betty repeatedly complained, she was bored stiff. The young doctor's heart went out to the youth of Force, who had no recreational choices besides the church-step card games and hitchhiking to movies. Above all, Hayes grew increasingly convinced that the filth and deterioration were killing people while the mining company looked on, unconcerned.

The mud-puddle streets nearly took the life of one of her patients when an ambulance, summoned from DuBois, sank down to its fenders. Hayes's car became mired, too, causing a dangerous delay. The community came up with a proposal to pave the road with "red dog," a mining waste product. The rose-colored gravel would cost Shawmut Mining nothing, and the miners offered to contribute the labor in their spare time. All that they and their doctor asked of Shawmut was the use of the company truck.

Management refused to cooperate. The company hadn't wanted Hayes here and wouldn't do anything to accommodate her needs, even in matters of life or death. Undaunted, Hayes made another request. This time, management had a bit of fun with her.

Among the many unfortunate architectural features of Force was the placement of coal sheds in its dwellings' front yards. This was for the company's convenience. Like other landlords, Shawmut had to provide coal, the main source of home heating in that era, to the tenants who'd dug it from the earth. Shoving it into front-yard shacks speeded delivery. Sagging under sloped roofs like the porches behind them, these large wooden structures were the first sight to greet visitors.

Hayes was determined to have the coal sheds moved from the front yards to the back ones. The miners don't seem to have joined her in this campaign. She reportedly wanted the placement changed because it was "dangerous for the children," but it's unclear what she meant by this. Presumably, children could lock one another up in the structures. They might also set them on fire, accidentally or purposely. Such dangers might have been mitigated or eliminated by moving the sheds to the back, where watchful mothers could see them from their kitchens. Placed in the front, beyond porches, they were almost in the road.

Or Hayes's request might have stemmed from concerns about "social hygiene," a subject she tackled in talks to groups of women and girls. The phrase was code at that time for sex education, including warnings about unplanned pregnancy and venereal disease. A roadside shed on a dark street might shelter an adolescent tryst or worse—newspaper accounts of sexual assaults in coal sheds were then not uncommon. Behind the houses, which were almost flush, they would have been less accessible to strangers.

However she expressed her concerns to Shawmut Mining, its officials pretended to agree. A truck was sent to the house next to hers, and carpenters got out, ostensibly to do the first moving job. Slowly they dismantled her neighbor's coal shed, and just as slowly, they reassembled it—again, in the front yard, just a few feet from its original site. The show was over.

The doctor had been pranked again or, more precisely, threatened.

"It is our property," Hayes was reportedly informed, "and if we want to put up coal sheds in the front yards, we'll put up coal sheds in the front yards."[2] The only published account of this incident doesn't specify the neighbor, who undoubtedly was in on the joke. Most likely it was David Bell Sr., the mine superintendent, whose wife had accidentally shot off their son's leg many years before. David Jr. was now a foreman in the mine, thanks to Leo, who couldn't save his limb but kept him alive.

Shawmut found time for such shenanigans despite its war-fueled production boom, interrupted by a nationwide miners' strike. The company's four mines were producing more than 600,000 net tons, 25 percent over their prewar levels. This activity ground to a halt in the spring of 1943. With coal operators and the UMWA unable to agree on a contract, John L. Lewis ordered his members to lay down their tools. As operations in Pennsylvania ceased, the editorial board of the DuBois paper wrote that "the continuance of idleness in the mines will prove a great source of inspiration to Hitler, Mussolini and company." That reflected the mood of the country, where other unions were holding to their no-strike pledge for the duration. When President Roosevelt threatened to send troops to the coalfields, Lewis countered, "You can't dig coal with bayonets."[3]

Soon Bell and Shawmut manager Frank Lambert had something else to do besides playing tricks with coal sheds. They were ordered to fly American flags over the Shawmut mines and post notices that the federal government was in possession. With the outcome of the war at stake, Roosevelt had put his Secretary of Interior, Harold L. Ickes, in charge of negotiations with the UMWA. The coal operators were to carry on with production and sales as usual, but as "operating managers" of the government.

In the end, the government handed Lewis a victory. For the first time, miners would get portal-to-portal pay, earning an hourly rate for time spent traveling underground between the mine entrance and the coal face. By the time the deal was struck, hundreds of thousands in Pennsylvania had stopped work for various durations. The Shawmut diggers seem to have stayed out relatively briefly. They worked 280 days that year, about the same as a year earlier.

With more coal to load on its freight cars, Shawmut's parent, the Pittsburg, Shawmut & Northern Railroad, also hummed with unaccustomed activity. That quickened the pace of life in St. Marys, where the Shawmut Line—only outsiders called it the PS&N—employed hundreds to run the trains, maintain the tracks, and fix the brakes. St. Marys was a railroad town, as evidenced by its gossip columns. When a local young woman returned from Kane with a diamond ring, it was compared to "a headlight on a Shawmut engine."

Hayes was also running at full throttle. In addition to her heavy schedule of appointments, there were always emergencies. In midsummer of 1943, a miner with a fractured skull was brought to her office. After a Saturday night out, he'd loosened his hold on a companion and fallen on the sidewalk. The circumstances probably reinforced Hayes's disdain for the bar in the Force Hotel. A few days later, she was summoned to Byrnedale Road early in the morning. A car had struck a miner who was walking to work in a heavy fog. She pronounced him dead.

That same year, there were seventeen serious accidents in Shawmut's four mines, about the same as in the previous two years. None were fatal, but all rendered the victims unable to work for sixty days or more. Many mine operators could count on the company doctor to contain disability payments by prematurely deeming injured men fit for work. Shawmut could expect no such collusion from Hayes.

There were gratifying moments, too. Hayes delivered scores of babies and dispensed antibiotics, still an awe-inspiring novelty. In 1920 the first physician in the Hayes family, her uncle Senes, watched six children in the same family die of diphtheria, standing by helplessly as their father dug their graves; no cemetery would risk contagion. But while medicine had advanced since her uncle's time as a company doctor, so had the threats to public health in Bennett's Valley. She worried most about the water, anxious that it would someday cause an outbreak. Perhaps, like Uncle Senes, she'd end up a witness to gravedigging, able to do nothing.

For now, she was a popular figure. As she arrived at patient homes, kids jumped on her car's running board, greeting her with cries of "Dr. Betty!" Their mothers would present her with fruit and vegetables grown in their victory gardens. Hayes accepted these offerings, probably with no intention of consuming them: the vegetable beds lay near oozing privies. With food rationed to conserve it for the troops, the people here were eager to join the home-front campaign, even if it meant planting in contaminated soil.

The nearby induction centers had been busy as well. By the middle of 1944, 85 of Force's 650 residents were in the military, and one had perished. Among those serving was Frank Skrzypek, a young coal loader whose mother had died, leaving his father to raise ten children alone. The youngest brother of Hayes's friend Martha Agosti, Lucian "Baker" Benevich, was a tail gunner, applying his country-boy sharpshooting skills against the Luftwaffe.

Two of Force's native sons distinguished themselves in Europe. A graduate of Weedville High, John Richards was a manager at a defense-plant job in Buffalo, New York, when he was drafted into the U.S. Army Air Corps. He rose swiftly to the rank of second lieutenant and earned a Bronze Star and the French Croix de Guerre for bravery. A local star even before his military decorations, Richards had been a crack player on the Force baseball team.

Another native son, Robert Paul Anderson, was a navigator on a bombing mission celebrated by newspapers in cinematic detail. The young miner was over Germany in a Flying Fortress, hit so badly that it couldn't

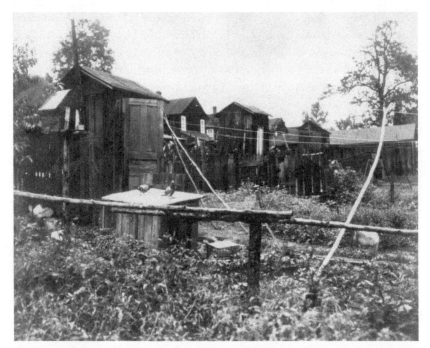

Outhouses drain into Force victory gardens. *Reproduced with permission from the Historical Society of Pennsylvania*

ascend beyond the treetops. Nevertheless, it dodged ground fire and fighter planes to bomb all its targets. Bob Anderson's crippled craft returned to base safely. However, his luck ran out a few months later. His aging parents were told that he was missing in action.

The president of Shawmut, John D. Dickson, had himself been an officer in World War I. But he apparently felt no special camaraderie with employees engaged in the current conflict. The local union leaders contended that draftees were entitled to their vacation pay. Management demurred, and the miners marched off without it. In the eyes of Dickson, the former army captain, they'd never be promoted from groundhogs.

This infuriated Hayes, who was passionately committed to honoring the local service members. She saw a chance to create something clean, lasting, and dignified in this almost comically deteriorating place. The residential section of Force might be called "the patch," but its young men were fighting for an America they'd seen in the movies.

Hayes began raising funds for a war monument. It was to be an honor roll, not a memorial, listing the names of area residents enlisted in the service. However, one would be marked with a gold star. Silvio Morelli, a miner, was the first casualty.

Hayes put together a committee to make this happen. Because miners would be asked to contribute toward the purchase of the $950 monument, the other members of the group were union leaders, leaving her the only woman. They would also need support from Shawmut. Plans called for a gala dance to follow the dedication ceremonies, with a live band amplified through a fire truck. A town of tenants couldn't undertake a project of this scope without their landlord's permission.

This time Shawmut came through, if not magnanimously, donating cement for the base of the monument. It also lent the use of its company truck, which it had so adamantly refused for the road-paving proposal. This was wartime. By this time, the Anderson boy had been found to be alive, but he was in a German prisoner-of-war camp. The Germans had also captured a son of the DeLullo family, owners of the independent grocery store inside the union hall. The mining concern couldn't refuse to help without seeming churlish or even unpatriotic.

The DuBois *Courier-Express* featured news of the committee's preparations on its front page, shoehorned into news of Allied victories in Italy and Burma. A band from St. Marys had been booked for the Saturday night dance. Speakers scheduled for the dedication included mine manager Frank Lambert and John Ghizzoni, an area resident who sat on the international board of the UMWA. A state assemblyman and the local district attorney rounded out the list, which was expected to expand.

Clouds and rain loomed over Bennett's Valley on the morning of June 3, 1944, but the weather was predicted to clear before the evening program. The forecast was a matter of acute interest there, as well as in Portsmouth, England, where the countdown to D-Day was secretly in progress.

Historical weather data doesn't specify whether the clouds lifted over the hills before Hayes, acting as mistress of ceremonies, unveiled the monument on the grounds of St. Joseph's Church. Other evidence suggests that the clouds had gone. Two thousand people from every town in the valley attended. Most were probably there to dance beneath the stars as music thundered from the fire engine.

Indeed, that was part of the idea behind this "gala," as its planners described it. Rationing, shortages, and worries about young people's mortality might be new to other parts of the country, but not here. As their physician, Hayes wanted these people to have some fun, to feel like they were worth it. Asked for an adjective to concisely describe her Aunt Betty,

Hayes's niece Nancy Huffman quickly volunteered "compassionate," also adding, "She was opinionated."[4]

Shawmut, uncharacteristically helpful in the planning, might have reverted to form with a last-minute stroke of malice. However, there are conflicting accounts of this. According to a Kane newspaper, the monument was dedicated by the four scheduled speakers, including Lambert, whom the paper described as a Punxsutawney resident. In fact, Lambert lived in St. Marys. But that wasn't the most serious error. As told by Hayes, Lambert was a no-show.

Three days after the gala, the weather cooperated again—this time at Normandy—and the Allies landed. As a magazine for veterans later phrased it, "On the very day some of the GIs from Force were sitting in landing craft off the coast of Normandy ready to go in for the D-Day assault, the company refused to attend the dedication ceremonies."[5] In war, as in peace, the company disappointed its towns.

Lambert would get another chance. Plans for another monument, more elaborate than the one in Force, were afoot. Hollywood, Mill Run, and Tyler also wanted an honor roll, to be located in Hollywood.

Hayes disapproved of inter-town rivalries, and the proposal smacked of one-upmanship. Still, she agreed to help the effort. She knew the families of Force best, but her practice also encompassed Hollywood and Mill Run. Her father's first job with Shawmut had been in Tyler, assisting his brother Senes.

Fundraising for the second monument renewed Hayes's links to the area union leaders, who worked in the Proctor No. 2 mine. Ted Challingsworth, although past the usual retirement age, was still active. He figured prominently in the monument proposal, as did a younger miner, Tony Guido. Two years before, they'd been instrumental in rousing the votes that let her fulfill her father's wishes. She owed her job to them.

Now she'd had enough of it. Not content with honoring the valley residents in the service, she wanted to see her own name on the honor roll. Even if she hadn't immersed herself in patriotic activities, the idea was to occur to her. Army and navy recruiters had descended on DuBois, where Hayes's work often took her. A Seabee float in the form of a ship plied the streets of Ridgway, DuBois, and Brockway, hoping to interest older men in the navy's civil engineering corps. Both the army and navy courted women for their Women's Army Auxiliary Corps (WAAC) and Women Accepted for Volunteer Emergency Service (WAVES), keeping the lights blazing at their DuBois recruitment centers into the evening hours.

Their efforts got a boost from the *Courier-Express*. In addition to its war-in-brief summaries and announcements of servicemen's birthdays, the paper began regularly publishing the names of area women who joined up. The onslaught continued on one Friday night at the Harris DuBois Theatre, where a short navy recruitment film, "Women in Blue," preceded the main feature.

Among the convinced was a Hayes relative. Single and twenty-three years old, Marguerite Garbarino had joined the WAVES. She was a granddaughter of Senes Hayes, the first of the family's coal-town physicians. Marguerite had no medical background, but she did share Hayes's independent streak. Rather than stay in Clarion, where she could work in her father's five-and-dime store, she had come to DuBois for a job in the Vulcan Soot Blower Company.

Now her name appeared in a patriotic advertisement sponsored by her former employer. Asking, "Do you want Nazi boots resounding on your home street . . . or little yellow men treating you like tyrants?" the ad promoted war bonds and listed an honor roll of Vulcan Soot Blower Company service members. Marguerite was grouped with the navy men, but a parenthetical note clarified her auxiliary status. As the first women besides nurses to serve in the U.S. military, WAACs and WAVES sometimes faced hostile questions about their femininity. They also had to endure marginal status as sex-segregated units assigned to noncombat zones.

For Marguerite's cousin Betty, on the other hand, opportunities in military service had broadened. In the spring of 1943, a new law allowed female medical doctors to be commissioned as officers in the army and navy's medical corps. Under previous rules, which had marginalized them into women's auxiliary service and prohibited them from treating men, only a handful had enlisted. As President Roosevelt put his signature to the law, women's advocates celebrated this culmination of a two-year struggle. But one leading proponent cautioned, "Now I'm hoping to see some women doctors commissioned. Only in that way will the law really mean anything."[6]

After several months, the navy put out a call for six hundred female medical officers. Someone like Hayes, who met all the requirements, would be commissioned as a lieutenant (junior grade) at minimum. She would be limited to shore duty within the continental United States, but otherwise would have the same status as the male doctors. Overseas service was allowed by the army, which, however, remained vague about how many women it intended to commission.

Hayes went through with it, submitting her application to the navy. This might seem an affront to her father's dying wish. Then again, as Betty understood it, or chose to understand it, the wish had a subordinating clause: Leo wanted one of his children to take care of the miners *until another qualified practitioner could take over.* And her father had made that wish before women could enlist as medical officers.

Betty Hayes was a prize catch for the navy recruiters. Of the estimated six thousand women licensed to practice medicine in the United States, only about one thousand were thought to be eligible for the military. Angering many who had fought for the new law, the navy narrowed the pool further by eliminating women with minor children. Single, childless, and a few years shy of thirty-five—the ceiling for nonspecialists—Hayes was the ideal candidate.

As Hayes would have known, her application required approval by the medical procurement and assignment board of the War Manpower Commission. Each state had such a board, charged with surveying the medical needs of communities and assigning medical practitioners to fill those needs. The aim was to address the scarcity of doctors in the civilian population produced by the call to duty.

The doctor shortage was acute not only in rural areas, but also in industrial zones with a heavy influx of factory workers. Outbreaks of influenza and tuberculosis were threatening to become health crises. There were proposals to suspend state licensing requirements and send physicians where they were most needed.

Yet the Pennsylvania board seemed loath to move doctors around the chessboard. A year after its establishment, it generated local news interest by transferring Dr. Alfred Dinert from small-town Lebanon to the tiny community of Dushore, more than one hundred miles north. In Lebanon, where Dinert was the house physician of Good Samaritan Hospital, the local paper noted, "It is the first reported transfer of a physician in northeastern Pennsylvania by the War Manpower Commission to overcome the civilian shortage of doctors due to army calls."[7]

In other states, too, the boards took their cues from the American Medical Association, which characterized such transfers as steps toward "socialized medicine." In moving Dinert, the board might have sought to improve its do-nothing image. If so, it had picked an easy target. Born in Poland and educated in Vienna, where he'd practiced for seven years, Dinert was a Jewish refugee. He'd just gotten settled in Lebanon, where his first child was born, when the transfer orders came. Not yet a citizen, he was in no position to complain.

The board rejected Hayes's application for a commission in the navy medical corps on the grounds that she was "essential." Never mind that the navy had issued a call for hundreds of women medical officers and that Hayes was one of the few qualified candidates. Rather than disturb any nonessential city doctors and send them to the wilds of Bennett's Valley, the procurement and assignment board neither procured a military medical officer nor assigned anyone to relieve a shortage. Because the board declined to do its job, Hayes was frozen to hers.[8]

If Hayes suspected Shawmut of helping to thwart her enlistment, the one brief press mention of the episode doesn't mention such suspicions. But Hayes firmly believed that the mining company had its fingers in state and local government, as she indicated on other occasions. The board would have called Shawmut for a reference, if nothing else. Given the physician shortage, the company wasn't likely to support her navy application.

That disappointment came in 1944, a difficult year for Hayes. She watched her mother make plans to leave Force while she remained stuck. In February, Anna Hayes and her son Vincent sued Leo's life insurance company. In April, a gossip item in a DuBois paper noted that Betty and Anna had been "business callers" in that city. Soon after that, Anna was granted a permit to build a home in Brockway.

All this suggests that the Hayes estate and the insurance company had reached a settlement. Meanwhile, Shawmut, always late in paying Leo, had yet to produce the thousands of dollars owed to him when he died. Now that she could afford to, Anna was making her exit.

For Betty, no amount of money could buy freedom. In fact, she was making a healthy income, as were many of her neighbors throughout the region. The strike settlement left miners earning nine or ten dollars a day. Some had annual incomes of $4,500, worth nearly $63,000 today. From her guaranteed income—the subsidy paid by Shawmut and the miners' paycheck deductions—Hayes earned slightly less than that. Fees paid by valley families unconnected with mining could potentially boost that figure to the equivalent of $117,000 today—or so claimed a Shawmut official, who was probably exaggerating. Hayes also treated indigent patients without expecting payment.

Around this time, a newspaper columnist in Hayes's area described company doctors as having "lucrative" practices. Assuming that was true, she still couldn't buy a replacement for herself. Called back from her adventures in Newfoundland and denied a chance to serve her country in uniform, she had little to look forward to other than mistress-of-ceremonies duties at the second monument dedication. This one wouldn't even include a dance. The Hollywood committee was planning an afternoon event of speakers followed by an accordion band.

At this point, an interesting figure entered Hayes's life. Ross H. Pentz was a prominent DuBois attorney. Middle-aged and of medium build, Pentz looked the stereotypical small-town lawyer. A photo, however, revealed a fierce look in the eyes behind his glasses. Under his shirtsleeves lurked a forearm tattoo, a souvenir of his colorful youth. In the first years of World War I, Pentz had left Princeton to drive an ambulance for the French army on the battlefields. Leaving the French for the U.S. Naval Air Force, he entered pilot training in those perilous early days of aviation, including a month of flight school in Miami.

But these Hemingway-esque beginnings were not to continue. Instead of piloting fighter aircraft over Europe, Pentz spent most of his war stateside, as an officer in a quartermaster corps. After the armistice, he wrestled for Princeton and earned a University of Pennsylvania law degree. Returning to DuBois, his birthplace, he joined his father and an older brother in the family law firm.

As Hayes confronted a future in Force without her mother, Ross Pentz at forty-six was also newly independent. After their father's death, his brother John had formed a new partnership with another attorney. Ross had done the same, practicing for the first time outside the family fold. Married with three children, the younger Pentz was deeply entrenched in civic affairs, active in veteran affairs and youth groups. He also represented several municipalities and was solicitor to the town council that granted Anna Hayes a building permit.

Approval of the permit came one month after Anna, in the company of Betty, made their business call to DuBois. Their destination might have been Pentz's East Long Street office, perhaps to complete paperwork. The Pentz and Hayes families had a long acquaintanceship. Back in the early 1920s, John Pentz had defended Gerald, the elder of Betty's two deceased brothers, for violating hunting rules by killing two deer in three days. The defense was unsuccessful, however. Leo ended up paying a fine of one hundred dollars, a staggering sum in those days, for his teenaged son's bravado. Betty was then a child, and Ross, eight years younger than John, was probably in law school.

At whatever point they met, Ross Pentz and Betty Hayes were to forge a formidable alliance. The navy's would-be flier and the rejected medical officer would find a war to win together.

Meanwhile, the world was still at war, but the collapse of Germany seemed imminent. Believing that the Allies were "over the hump," tens of thousands of Americans were leaving war-related jobs for better offers. Alarmed by what it called "over-optimism," the federal government took charge of job referrals in many areas, replacing corporate personnel offices and union hiring halls. The miners of Bennett's Valley were deemed essential, like Hayes. And like her, they were frozen to their jobs.

By the spring of 1945, Anna's house was taking shape in Brockway. The mother's looming departure might have prepared the daughter for a desperate gamble. Too busy to prepare her own meals or even hang up her clothes, Hayes must have viewed the future with apprehension. Around this time Hayes, spattered in sewage, was delivering a baby. She'd slipped in one of the open drains that passed for roads in Force.

It was the last straw. On April 15, 1945, three days after the death of Franklin D. Roosevelt, Hayes resigned—or more precisely, announced her intention to resign. The letter she sent to Shawmut has not survived, but her subsequent comments make clear that it was conditional. She set her terms for staying in her post: the coal company would have to provide its communities with decent water supplies, some efforts at sewage disposal, streets, and streetlights. She also set Friday, June 15, as the date she planned to depart if her terms were not met. Shawmut had two months to find a qualified replacement for her.

There was no reply to her letter, just dead silence. The mining company also failed to notify the War Manpower Commission of the resignation, disregarding federal guidelines that had gone into effect with the national job freeze. With the commission's U.S. Employment Service now in control of job referrals, the mining company needed to inform it of the impending vacancy. Instead, the resignation "slumbered in the company files," as one journalist reported.[9]

Shawmut didn't take Hayes seriously. When the company finally notified the commission of her resignation, "I suppose they took it for granted that we had accepted it," Lambert said. He set the record straight: "We haven't acted on it."[10] If Hayes suspected Shawmut of having thwarted her navy plans, such suspicions were reasonable. Dismissing her resignation letter, Dickson, the company president, wrote, "The plain truth is that because of some personal and selfish ambitions of Dr. Hayes, she demanded to be released from her duties. If we had consented, it would have deprived our employees of needed medical services."[11] Dickson seemed to think he could keep Hayes working against her will.

But she knew she had the upper hand, as Lambert might have learned from his colleague from the company snoop, F. J. Erich. The industrial detective's tasks could have taken him to the misnamed Hollywood where the construction of the monument was still underway, with cement and lumber donated by Shawmut and hauled by a company truck. Germany and Italy had surrendered, but many area residents were in the Pacific. The honor roll of men and women in the service had swelled to 113, with three killed in action.

Slated to be mistress of ceremonies at the late-July dedication, Hayes might have told the committee that she couldn't guarantee her appearance. Ted Challingsworth, head of the Hollywood union local, would have been alarmed. A volunteer firefighter, Challingsworth was likely a member of the Proctor No. 2 mine rescue team. Such teams worked closely with physicians after rockfalls and other accidents, administering first aid and bringing the injured to the surface.

Still not thrilled with their woman doctor, as suggested by later events, the Proctor No. 2 miners were not wholly trustworthy as Hayes allies. Challingsworth officially sided with her against management, but not as vocally as his Proctor No. 1 counterparts. It's also unclear if the opinions of Challingsworth, now in his late sixties, still carried the weight they once did with the rank and file

Still, no miner—particularly a rescuer—could share Shawmut's sanguine view of Hayes's resignation. Nobody wanted to go into the pits without a doctor handy. In the first half of 1945, there had been two serious accidents in the old Proctor No. 1 mine and three in newer No. 2, which hired fewer men but used more power equipment. Through the "pussyfoot" Erich or other channels, the men made their agitation known.

The weather grew warmer, but in Force people still closed their windows at night. In summer, the place became a "stinking gob pile," as one editorial elegantly put it.[12] There were also the usual cases of illnesses caused by the contaminated water. Mining folk often called this "summer dysentery," but as the filthy privies deteriorated further, Hayes feared an outbreak of typhoid fever.

Twenty-four hours before Hayes was scheduled to leave, she got a phone call. It was Lambert, asking her to give him another month—not to meet her terms, but to find a replacement. He claimed that the company had made strenuous efforts to find another doctor, but he needed more time. In fact, Shawmut had done nothing. After neglecting to list the vacancy with the federal employment service, it had failed to advertise in the *Journal of the American Medical Association*, a leading resource for physician employment.

Having heard nothing from the War Manpower Commission, and as a member of the AMA, Hayes probably knew that Lambert was lying. His phone call revealed that she had the company over a barrel. It also indicated that they might make the lies true by searching for a replacement in earnest. As much as she'd wanted to leave, she was now determined to stay. She saw how much she might accomplish by doing so.

She laid out the situation to the union leaders. Delegates from the three locals sat on a miners' committee, the rural equivalent of an urban central labor council. Occasionally, they met with management to discuss issues of common concern. Ironically, the committee had requested such a meeting the previous year, not to discuss the filth of the water, but to complain that there was not enough of it. A dry spell had left the towns parched—"something for which the Company was in no way responsible," wrote Dickson.[13]

So informed by Dickson's intermediaries, the miners' committee dropped the matter, made moot when the rains came. The experience vindicated Dickson's belief that workers could be persuaded to see things from his own, very reasonable viewpoint. Prepared to throw up his hands again, he had no objection to hearing the miners out. He understood that the request for this meeting was "inspired," as he put it, by Dr. Hayes and her unhappiness about sanitation. Dickson also knew that sanitation fell outside the bounds of the UMWA contract.

What's more, there was a job freeze on. If Hayes or the miners expected to work somewhere else, they'd need Dickson to sign a release form. The war had given him a tremendous amount of power.

Arrangements were made for a July 2 meeting with the labor committee. Dickson's mine manager, Lambert, would be present, but Dickson himself would remain north of the Pennsylvania–New York border. However, his vice president, P. B. McBride, was to attend and report back. For all Dickson's professed confidence, he knew the men were agitated; otherwise, he wouldn't have sent the lofty McBride to meet with the miners.

Across the nation, women were being pressured to leave the labor force and hand their jobs to veterans. But in Bennett's Valley, a woman's pending resignation had called all parties to the table. Later, ruing his part in it, Dickson saw her as an enchantress who'd bewitched all parties. He wrote that she was "not unlike . . . the sirens of old," adding, "Had we all, miners and company representatives alike, made use of wax as did Ulysses, we would have most certainly avoided this most unfortunate position in which we find ourselves."[14]

With or without wax earplugs, Dickson had no intention of listening to Hayes. But she was about to turn up the volume.

3

THE ULTIMATUM

The vice president of Shawmut, Peter B. McBride, was a "very big man and from appearance might become a very tough gentleman if sufficiently provoked," in the words of a journalist who took care not to test his hypothesis.[1] Tall and barrel-shaped, with dark brows and a broad face, McBride looked like he had spent his life in the mines; however, he'd never needed to use his brawn. His formidable powers flowed from other sources.

His older sister Mayme, a one-time clerk for the Shawmut rail line, had brought Pete into the business, where he soon rose above her. Starting as chief clerk, he became the auditor and controller for the Shawmut interests while still in his youth. Now in his mid-fifties, Pete McBride was still single. He lived with Mayme and another sister in the large brick mansion inherited from their father, an Irish-born watchmaker who did well in the jewelry business. Like the father, many of Pete's ten siblings were accomplished musicians. Three were organists at Catholic churches, and the eldest played violin at nightclubs until a fall down a boarding-house staircase cut his life short.

Pete found a different path to local fame. After presiding over the St. Marys town council as burgess, he'd been elected mayor in the mid-1930s. While in office he took part in a Democratic Party parade, escorting a member of Congress in a car followed by a braying donkey. A searchlight affixed to the roof of the McBride home illuminated the procession. Subsequently, he was elected an associate judge of Elk County, running unopposed on both the Democratic and Republican tickets and serving until 1941.

McBride had done all this while simultaneously holding the second-highest office at both the PS&N Railroad and Shawmut Mining—like the bar owner in a classic Western movie who, it turns out, is also the judge and sheriff. Too important a man to concern himself with the day-to-day operations of the mine, he left those to the mine manager, Frank Lambert, who in turn depended on Dave Bell, mine superintendent and Hayes's longtime neighbor. Now sixty-one, McBride had known the doctor since she was a child.

On the first Monday of July 1945, all three sat opposite the miners' committee and Dr. Hayes. If minutes were taken, they haven't survived. We have only Dickson's account—based on his subordinates' report to him and described in a letter—and a magazine piece based on interviews with Hayes and the miners.

Neither version mentioned the meeting location, but it was probably in St. Marys, where the offices of the PS&N Railroad and its mining subsidiaries sprawled over four floors in two buildings. An army of white-collar workers toiled in these environs, although the need for so many of them was mysterious. One of Lambert's sons, recently added to the payroll, was rarely seen.

As for the miners at the meeting, Dave Bell was probably the only manager who knew them by name. No list of the miners' committee members present has survived. Tony Coccimiglio, president of both the Force and Byrnedale locals, was almost certainly there with his brother-in-law, Norman Winkler, and Norman's father, Frank. Among the others who likely attended were Bill Agosti, who had defended Hayes against sexual harassment, and Ted Challingsworth, president of the Hollywood local. These were men willing to expose themselves to the many retributions available to the company, which paid their salary, owned their houses, and manipulated the local government.

It was an extraordinary session. On Dickson's orders, the executives were meeting with the doctor, as well as the men, on a matter not covered by the labor contract. The managers had every reason for confidence. Although Japan wasn't yet defeated, the newspapers were heralding a postwar period of sleek new homes brimming with washing machines and dishwashers. However, the miners had been made no such promises. In the latest wage negotiations, the bituminous coal operators flatly rejected a United Mine Workers of America demand for better housing. Management had even nixed a plan to have a committee explore the issue.

As Dickson later wrote with his pretentious literary flourishes, "Our Mr. Lambert and Mr. McBride graciously agreed to attend such meeting, although from a technical standpoint there was not the slightest requirement for them so to do [sic]." Things rapidly grew less gracious. Hayes did most of the speaking and, according to Dickson, "There seems to be no limit to the abuses in which the Doctor indulged, and her demands were, to say the least, fantastic."[2] If he meant that they required imagination, he wasn't far from the truth.

Hayes sketched out a vision of mining towns governed by their residents. To McBride, who was there, and Dickson, who heard about it, the proposal was outlandish. Yet, Hayes didn't begin at this point, nor did she necessarily expect to arrive there. The meeting began, quite literally, with a nuts-and-bolts proposal.

The miners' committee had also looked into the cost of a water and sewage system. A water company had worked out a quote for piping in water from Penfield, six miles from Force. For $25,000, they could have fresh water and a sewer system. There were also calculations for providing indoor bathrooms. Those who wanted them offered to do the labor themselves.

Flush with wartime cash, many miners had already been painting and decorating the interiors of their homes. Some had even installed new sinks, though no water ran from the taps. They were willing to pay for water and sewers through rent increases.

The Shawmut managers would have none of it. They also warned that they'd arrest anyone involved in such construction for trespassing if the work proceeded without their consent. For this, they could count on Erich, their one-man police force.

Undeterred, Hayes presented what she called her "blueprint" for a community where health could thrive. Once again, she demanded paved streets. Garbage must be collected, not thrown on a festering heap. Foundations should be laid under houses, and retaining walls built to halt front-yard erosion.

There was no money for this, the managers said, bringing Hayes to her next point.

She envisioned towns that would identify their needs and—unimpeded by Shawmut—raise money and donate labor to meet them. Her "fantastic" plan (in Dickson's words) called for incorporating communities that could govern themselves.[3] When McBride threatened to arrest plumbing contractors for trespassing, Hayes countered, "I charge the company with deliberate obstructionism. . . . Why don't you build a fence around the town and call yourself Lord McBride? This is a tyranny as bad as the colonists were subjected to, and someone ought to throw a Boston Tea Party."[4]

Continuing at full throttle, Hayes demanded the closure of the Force Hotel and the company stores. Force's priest, Reverend Francis Ferrara, and Bishop John Mark Gannon of the Erie diocese also came in for a drubbing. The product of a Catholic secondary-school education, Hayes may have unsuccessfully sought support from these clergymen. McBride, a fellow Catholic and brother of three church organists, apparently viewed these attacks as heresy.

Dickson, an Episcopalian, professed to share his underling's shock. In outrage, real or pretended, he complained that the doctor's demands "ranged anywhere from the insistence that we take steps to incorporate our mining communities to the removal of the local dominie. In fact," he confided to a correspondent, "aspersions were even cast upon the Bishop of the Diocese." In the Dicksonian version of these events, "Mr. McBride made a gentlemanly attempt to refute some of these baseless charges, but was only met with further abuses."[5] Almost six feet tall and weighing 190 pounds, McBride saw himself as the doctor's helpless victim.

It's unclear whether Hayes had intended to go quite this far. At least one of the miners told the press later that he didn't necessarily agree with the whole scope of her demands. She herself later clarified one point, denying she had ever insisted on indoor bathrooms. It was possible to construct sanitary outhouses—the Works Progress Administration had done it for years—and she didn't want to seem desirous of "luxuries." But she never deviated from her overarching theme. Fix-it projects would not be enough. She wanted "genuine community life" in Force and its neighbors.[6] And except for the bathroom bit, she never took back a word she said. She saw no sense in treating patients while their environment was endangering them, physically and mentally.

Her speech made quite an impression on Frank Lambert, who knew Hayes was well-liked in the mining towns. Only a few years before, he had failed in his effort to replace the doctor with someone more likely to be compliant. He also knew the miners, and he was amazed that they let her speak this way.

Lambert was floored by the support the men gave her, as his subsequent comments made clear. McBride, on the other hand, saw chinks in the armor. Recording the latter's impressions, Dickson wrote, "To the credit of the Mine Committee, I'm happy to say that they did not indulge in the tirades and the unwarranted charges hurled against our Company and its officials which were indulged in by Dr. Hayes. In fact, they openly stated to our representatives that they did not and could not condone many of the charges and would not be a party to some of the demands."[7]

Lambert, sensing solidarity, and McBride, smelling fear, would both prove to be right. McBride's antennae could have picked up discomfort from the Hollywood delegation. Ted Challingsworth was immersed in plans for the upcoming monument dedication. Civic and business leaders were expected to speak. For the miners of Hollywood and its neighboring hamlets, this wasn't an apt time for conflict.

Still, something had come over the miners, who for decades had lived in what one journalist called "supine submission."[8] Lambert sensed they were taking their cues from Hayes. He felt the temperature rising in the room.

Dickson's absence left a convenient excuse to end the meeting. Mc-Bride and Lambert could scorn the proposals and declare them impossible, but they couldn't say anything definite. The big men in town were mere second lieutenants to their captain. They'd have to get back to the miners. No date for the next meeting was fixed. Not then. Not in the doctor's presence.

Even the status of Hayes's resignation was left hanging, as it had been for so long. She said she would stay another year, but only if sanitary conditions were improved. McBride told her he'd have to run that by Dickson.

At his aerie in Wellsville, far away from the song of the "siren," Dickson got an earful. His interpretation, or so he wrote in a letter, was that Hayes's motives were purely selfish. All she wanted was the acceptance of her resignation so that she could leave her job. The sanitation issue was just a smokescreen.

Dickson expressed certainty that the problems were her invention. "I am reliably informed that up until a month ago we received no complaints whatsoever from our miners relative to sanitary conditions, or the water supply," he wrote.[9] His letter consumed several sheets of stationery headed by the grinning groundhog with pick and helmet, content to live in dirt. He added that Hayes had never raised issues about sanitation until she asked to resign. Considering her previous requests for road paving and the moving of coal sheds, as well as her reports of suspected typhoid cases, this is unlikely.

Confident that any reasonable person, including the recipient of his letter, would see his point, Dickson presented the wartime economic boom as a financial calamity. "The expenditure of any moneys by our Company at this time is an impossibility," he wrote, assigning responsibility to the worldwide conflict. He said his workforce had decreased by nearly half since "slightly before the Pearl Harbor episode," resulting in "an inordinate loss of production." As with Hayes, Dickson saw selfishness and disloyalty in the men who'd left his employment. "At least 60% of these losses involve employees who sought employment in so-called war plants . . . where promises of higher wages and less work were the order of the day," he wrote.

The former Captain Dickson, a veteran of the First World War, neglected to note that the other 40 percent had left to serve, and sometimes die, in the armed forces. Nor did he mention that the war had increased rail business on the Shawmut Line. The railroad's only reason for existence was to haul coal from mines owned by Shawmut and other operators, and those "so-called war plants" he'd maligned were clamoring for coal. Indeed, 1941 had produced record income for the railroad.

In his correspondence, Dickson is dismissive of Hayes, but, in reality, she rattled him. He convinced himself that she had to be removed from the equation. Then he could reach some kind of agreement with the men, who had never been this troublesome before.

Through McBride and Lambert, Dickson arranged a second talk— with at least some miners—to be conducted without the doctor present and likely without her knowledge. Though probably brief, it was held in person rather than by telephone. Dickson left a written record of the date, July 14, a Saturday. He didn't note the location, most likely St. Marys.

Not truly a meeting, the July 14 encounter was a clandestine conference about scheduling a meeting. Dickson wrote that he'd been present at this talk, but that's probably untrue. Months later, Tony Coccimiglio would face Dickson in a federal courtroom and testify that he'd never seen him before. Moreover, it's doubtful that Dickson would have bothered to leave his western New York home, particularly on a weekend. He relegated these colonial matters to Lord McBride, who seemed to relish intimidating people.

The only item on the agenda was resolved. A second meeting between labor and management on sanitation was scheduled for the following Wednesday, July 18. Everyone left understanding one thing: Dr. Hayes could not be present. Dickson wrote that she "had disqualified herself from participating in any conference at which friendly relations could be maintained." According to Dickson, the miners readily agreed to this non-negotiable condition. Not a whiff of dissent was heard from them. All seemed harmonious as they headed home, ready to meet openly on Wednesday.

The next few hours marked a fateful change of course. Whether from fear or just playing for time, some men had betrayed Hayes by agreeing to cut her out. But on that same Saturday, she had some news to announce to them. Shawmut had finally accepted her resignation. No one from the company had bothered to contact her. She'd heard about it from the War Manpower Commission.

She was no longer the company physician. On Monday, the men would be going into the mines without any doctor available for miles around. What's more, she was serious about exploring her options elsewhere. That would leave the men, women, and children of Bennett's Valley's eleven towns without medical care.

Determined to vanquish the siren—half-monster and half-woman—Dickson had given Hayes a cudgel instead.

It was a busy weekend in Bennett's Valley. Within hours of the meeting in St. Marys, Dickson got a call. The miners who'd agreed to the Wednesday meeting had reversed themselves. It was off.

Other meetings were held, families were consulted, and votes were taken. Locals 97, 6397, and 851 had to decide whether to follow Hayes off the job. Calls were made to Ross Pentz, who agreed to represent the miners' committee. He thought the men might qualify for unemployment benefits if they stopped work. State law protected employees from being compelled to work under unsafe conditions, and mining without a doctor on hand was anything but safe.

Sensing, or perhaps knowing through informants, that some miners were prepared to work around her, Hayes made another thing clear. She'd stay another year, or until a suitable replacement was found for her. However, her promise stood only if the miners solidly backed her—there could be no side deals and no settling for token concessions. They had to be all in, all of them together. She put it very simply: If the men returned to work, "she'd take her bag and leave," as Coccimiglio later testified.[10]

On Monday, trains whistled past the three towns without stopping. There was no coal to be loaded. None of the 350 miners employed at the Proctor mines had shown up for work.

4

THE SIRENS SING

The DuBois *Courier-Express*, once so interested in Betty Hayes's male houseguest, regularly covered local strikes and reprinted United Press stories about national ones. Yet weeks had passed since Hayes's resignation had sparked a work stoppage, and the paper hadn't written a single line about it.

That's what the miners were calling it: a work stoppage, not a strike. Hayes referred to it as a protest. If it were a strike, the United Mine Workers of America would have had to take a position on it, either authorizing it or ordering the men back to work. But throughout July, the UMWA stayed out of it. The union's top official in the region would later say he knew nothing about it until much later.

That was a lie, as anyone from the area would have suspected. The union locals in Force, Byrnedale, and Hollywood were part of the UMWA's District 2, whose gray-haired president, James Mark, lived in DuBois. Like all district presidents, Mark was a trusted appointee of the notoriously distrustful John L. Lewis. At the Union Building in the town of Clearfield, southeast of Force, Mark received letters from the presidents of the locals in his central Pennsylvania territory. Ordinary miners also wrote to him about everyday concerns. Whether typed neatly or scrawled in pencil, many of these letters got a response. There was no chance that Mark wouldn't know what was happening in Force.

Contrary to the district president's later protestations of ignorance, Mark wrote to Dickson three days after the miners laid down their tools, asking him to resume talks about unsanitary conditions in Force with the miners' committee, Dr. Hayes, "and any other interested persons."[1]

While awaiting a response from Dickson in New York, Mark had sent a board member to represent the district at the dedication ceremony for the war monument in Hollywood. Compared to its counterpart in Force, held a year earlier on the brink of D-Day, it was a quiet affair. The Proctor No. 2 mine was silent. A few hundred people listened as Judge F. Cortez Bell made a short speech, quoting President Truman, who said that the goal of the war was "a peaceful life."

The marble monument was unveiled. Engraved with the names of 111 service members from Hollywood, Tyler, and Mill Run, it had been purchased with funds raised by the miners. Hayes, the mistress of ceremonies, thanked each participant and pointedly noted Shawmut's donations of sand and cement. Her message was clear: No one from management was present.

The *Courier-Express* featured the event on the front page of its July 23, 1945, edition. Yet the article neglected to mention the work stoppage in Hollywood and the doctor's extraordinary role in it. While regularly running news of coal strikes elsewhere, the DuBois paper ignored the strife in its own backyard.

After the closing prayers, the doctor and the miners had to consider their next steps. In addition to filing unemployment claims, Ross Pentz sent a notice of Hayes's resignation and the resulting work stoppage to the Solid Fuels Administration, the federal agency in charge of wartime controls on coal production, pricing, and distribution.

No immediate reply came from Harrisburg. But in New York, a few days after the monument dedication, Dickson responded to the union's request that Hayes be admitted to the bargaining table. It was then that he produced his letter charging Hayes with resigning for purely selfish reasons and ensorcelling men with her siren song. Attempting a puckish jest, he essentially charged her with witchcraft.

The recipient of these erudite witticisms was none other than James Mark, the UMWA district president. Now sixty-eight, Mark had left school for the mines at age eleven. Born in Scotland and raised in Pennsylvania, he signed his name with a big scrawl. But Mark was an important figure in labor, often quoted in the papers, and Dickson liked dealing with others of his own rank. Mark was, after all, a man. The industrialist was confident he could convert him to an anti-Hayes ally.

In his letter, Dickson made a concession, saying he might be willing to sit down with the miners and discuss one or two matters regarding sanitation: "I think it will be admitted by all concerned that they could not be properly brought up under our contract, but I am not one who desires to be too technical when the relations of employer and employee are involved."[2]

One point, however, was non-negotiable. Any negotiations would have to occur "without the benefit of the presence of Dr. Hayes," who, "by her conduct at a former meeting . . . had disqualified herself from participating in any conference at which friendly relations could be maintained."

Mark made no immediate reply, and the correspondence went on hiatus.

By now, the miners had missed checks for two weeks with no word from the unemployment board; however, there were stirrings from the state health department, which finally responded to the reports of well contamination and suspected typhoid in Force. Late in July, near the end of a work week, Pentz's notices bobbed to the surface at the health department's headquarters in Harrisburg. A district sanitary engineer was dispatched to Force.

The engineer, M. J. Barrick, was a familiar figure at area town council and commerce board meetings. He advised on the construction of municipal swimming pools and other large and costly public projects. He had the authority to inform municipalities that they must find funds to construct sewage plants or other facilities to comply with state law.

Barrick worked at a district office in Williamsport, more than one hundred miles east of Force. His job often involved travel, but this appointment was scheduled suddenly and on a Sunday. The health department's sanitary division had a representative closer at hand in DuBois, but that inspector was on vacation. Thus inconvenienced, Barrick found himself meeting with Hayes, a person of no authority. She wasn't even the company doctor anymore.

Clouds had hung over the valley for several days. Temperatures stayed in the eighties with daily thunderstorms or showers. The mud and stink of Force were in full summer bloom. Hayes must have been filled with hope as she prepared to show the state health department representative around. Barrick was a veteran engineer, trained by the military during the First World War. Moreover, he had the results of the private lab tests. People were drinking their own sewage. Surely the health department would see the danger of typhoid.

Instead, the engineer treated this Sunday disruption as a false alarm. Force was no worse off than other mining towns, he informed Hayes, obviously thinking she should have known better. He did nothing other than to leave her with this advice: "But doctor, why don't you wait until an epidemic breaks out before you kick up all this fuss?"[3]

Those words, recounted by her in press interviews and sworn testimony—and never challenged by Barrick or his employer—inspired

Hayes's next move. If the state couldn't be moved to action, then the public would have to be moved by her story. Hayes had to sit down with someone who knew the news business to do something she generally avoided: talk about herself.

On the afternoon of July 31, news of the Third Fleet's attack on Japan shared the *Pittsburgh Press*'s front page with the photo of Hayes. With her waved hair and button earrings, she smiled beneath a headline, "Woman Doctor, Miners Quit in Fight to Clean Up Coal Towns." The piece began with an intensely personal focus on Hayes, her desire to "do things" to better the miners' lives, and her father's legacy. Speaking for Shawmut, Lambert said the company wouldn't accept the private lab's findings without state confirmation. He said improvements were "not possible at this time," adding that finding a replacement for Hayes was "well-nigh impossible."[4]

Written by a stringer based in DuBois—perhaps a staffer for the *Courier-Express*—the story proved instantly appealing. Abbreviated and without the photo, the same piece ran in Pittsburgh's evening paper, the *Sun-Telegraph*. The United Press picked it up. Some other papers, mostly in Pennsylvania, ran a short version.

It was also noticed at the Capitol in Harrisburg. By the end of the business day, state health officials had located Paul Heitzenrater, their DuBois-based field inspector. The father of three was ordered to cut short his family vacation and head to Force immediately.

This time, Hayes brought a group of miners with her, as well as the reporter. It was another soggy day, too rainy for Heitzenrater to take water samples, but he toured the malodorous landscapes with his hosts. The local *Pittsburgh Press* stringer was also on hand, taking notes as Heitzenrater repeatedly muttered, "Pretty bad. It isn't very pretty." Offered a drink of murky water from one of the wells by miner Joe Shadick, the state inspector declined. "I wouldn't take a drink of that on a bet," he said, and Shadick replied, "Neither would I."[5]

Praising Hayes's skills as a doctor, the miners also reiterated their refusal to go into the mines without "a doctor" close by. Mindful of the argument underpinning their unemployment claim, they didn't insist on Hayes's rehiring, but their meaning was obvious.

Those quotes ran the next day in the *Press*, in the first story filed from Force. But as August began, a parade of big-city journalists headed for the hills. They were eager to see the young woman who, Lambert said, had whipped the miners into a "white heat" and "organized them like the thirteen colonies" until they were "ready to stage another Boston tea party."[6]

But widespread attention had drawbacks. Hayes and her allies were no longer able to control the narrative. As the month began, the "white heat" quote, with its suggestion of lasciviousness, ran in a Toronto paper under the heading, "Miners Excited Over Bathrooms." Some clever headline writer saw an opportunity to exploit stereotypes of rural people while trivializing life-threatening sanitation issues.

More seriously, the Pennsylvania Department of Health began minimizing the situation. There was a lot to minimize. State testing, still ongoing, had found human-waste contamination in five of seven wells tested in Force, Hollywood, and Byrnedale, as well as Weedville, which was not company-owned.

There would be no more expressions of sympathy from Heitzenrater in newsprint. On August 1, he met with Shawmut officials, and his superiors took charge of the messaging. A plan was devised to repair privies, clean wells, and disinfect soil and water. In the meantime, boil-water notices would be posted.

In other words, all the towns needed was a good cleanup.

Caught off guard by Hayes's sudden celebrity, the health department had regained its balance. As Heitzenrater continued to sample water and putter around privies, press questions were referred to Dr. J. Moore Campbell, a deputy secretary of health and director of the department's Bureau of Health Conservation. More adept with the press than Lambert, Campbell was eager to protect his agency's image and not unduly concerned with the truth. Asked why a state sanitary engineer had visited Force and done nothing, Campbell said the engineer hadn't understood that the complaint referred to wells. Obviously, that was a falsehood.

The state health official became not only Shawmut's ally but its mouthpiece. Contacted by the Associated Press's Harrisburg reporter about Force, Campbell said, "It's practically impossible for the company to extend water lines to the mining hamlets which are several miles from the source of supply."[7] The state was taking the company's position, nearly word for word.

For the United Press, Campbell summed up conditions in Force as "no better or no worse than can be found in most communities," and said there was "little possibility" of a typhoid outbreak if "ordinary precautions" were taken. "The problem is a minor one and can be corrected," he said.[8] He had solved one problem, at least. As news of Force spread worldwide, the *Courier-Express* in DuBois broke its seventeen-day silence about the work stoppage. Reluctant to take sides openly, the paper seized on the remarks of Dr. Campbell, presumably a disinterested third party. Printing the

UP piece on its front page, the DuBois paper framed it as a public-health message rather than a delayed report on labor unrest. A few sentences preceding the wire story assured readers in the affected towns that the state would fix matters "rapidly." In the meantime, the paper wrote, there was "little" danger of disease. Boiling water was just an "extra safeguard."[9]

Hayes was livid. Campbell, a fellow physician, got under her skin in a way that Shawmut never did, at least when the battle was confined to words.

Shawmut had found a powerful ally. But as Campbell spoke to reporters in Harrisburg, mining families in Force were welcoming three notepad-toting visitors into their homes. The kettles were on, at full boil.

Elaine Kahn and Julia Shawell came to Force from the state's largest cities, Kahn from the AP's Pittsburgh office, and Shawell from the *Philadelphia Record*. They were a study in contrasts. Kahn, nearly twenty-three, was a recent graduate of the University of Pittsburgh, passionate about sportswriting. Shawell, old enough to be Kahn's mother, was a former film and drama critic with rouged cheeks and a taste for fur wraps, turbans, and corsages.

Judy Shepard had come the farthest. Even younger than Kahn, she had some of Shawell's experience. Expelled from the University of Wisconsin for flouting curfew rules that applied only to women, she'd been at the *New York Post* since age seventeen. In three years she'd made the leap from cub reporter to correspondent.

The war made Hayes irreplaceable, and it gave her a chance to tell her story. A newsroom survey conducted a year earlier found that eight thousand male reporters had joined the armed forces, replaced almost entirely by women. No longer confined to the cultural desk and women's pages, female journalists were writing about politics, business, and train wrecks. Still, barriers remained.

"I covered everything," Kahn said years later about her job for the AP, "and this made me infinitely superior—or, at least, I thought I was superior—to any other women who worked on Pittsburgh papers." Even in wartime, she said, each of her city's dailies had just one woman on the news desk, expecting her to present a uniquely feminine angle. Known derisively as a sob sister, this individual wrote "about servicemen's wives and that sort of thing," Kahn said.[10]

Understandably, Kahn wanted nothing of this. She'd broken barriers by becoming the first woman sports editor at her campus paper. As such, she regularly received mail addressed to "Mr. Elaine Kahn." Some people were quicker to believe that Elaine might be a man's name than that a woman could describe football games play by play. Reporting on professional sports for the AP—as well as steel strikes and presidential visits—"I couldn't go into the dressing room, but I never missed a story," she said.[11]

Yet Kahn took a somewhat sob-sisterly approach in reporting on Force, asking wives of the miners for their opinions of Hayes. Wives' comments comprised only a small portion of the AP story she filed from Force, which ran in papers across the nation. But in an era when films and books played up tensions between wives and secretaries, headlines like "Housewives Holding Fast for Cleanup" and "Wives Backing Up Miners Who Demand Sanitation" eliminated Hayes from any suspicion of home-wrecking.

The three journalists found the doctor immersed in domesticity. Hayes was rolling rugs, crating dishes, and taking pictures off the wall of her house. She told the reporters that she was planning to leave "as soon as I can" because of the "intolerable" conditions. No destination was specified. Hayes was probably packing these items for her mother, whose new house in Brockway was nearing completion. But as Anna Hayes looked on—and gave a quote to a reporter—neither she nor Betty corrected the impression that the rugs and dishes would follow the doctor to parts unknown.

New to the public stage but accustomed to dealing with Shawmut, Hayes knew that her bargaining power was strongest—with management as with the miners—when her departure seemed imminent. Anyway, it was true enough that she was in an unsettled state, wanting to flee but feeling the tug of responsibility. She'd promised the men to stay as long as they lined up behind her, but recent events had shaken her resolve.

Finally, the state health authority had come to Force, only to dismiss the gravity of the health threat and release Shawmut from any liability. Moreover, Campbell had misrepresented the company as a willing partner in any required cleanup while it hadn't even posted boil-water notices. As always in the towns that it owned, Shawmut wrote its own laws.

This time, though, others were watching. As Heitzenrater collected water samples for testing in Harrisburg, members of the miners' committee accompanied him. They stopped by the big doc's house to talk to the women reporters. Pens scratched paper as Bill Agosti declared, "We'll hold out as long as we have to."[12] For the visiting journalists, this was not just another strike story. In their hands, Force became a real-life version of the New York World's Fair exhibits that Hayes had seen six years earlier. This backward hellhole was a community of Americans, striving for democracy, progress, and all the conveniences of the World of Tomorrow.

August 1 was a busy day in Force. Members of mining families, including some related to strike leaders, appeared in photos highlighting the town's deprivations. These were obviously posed. Boys pictured fishing in a sewage-filled ditch couldn't hide their grins. Miners with pressed shirts and pomaded hair gathered on the steps of an outhouse—surely not their usual meeting place. One miner, stripped to the waist and grinning, splashed himself with rainwater collected in a metal washtub. "This is the only means they have to wash after leaving mining pits," the caption said, although with the strike on, no one had been in the pits that day.

Staged or not, the pictures demonstrated the broad support behind Hayes. Risking the ridicule of city dwellers, the families of Force put themselves on display. Distributed by the AP, the photos were widely reprinted, including by the *New York Times*. Hayes was no longer the exclusive focus. "There is not one factor here that constitutes a community," she told Kahn, referring to the filth, the nonpotable water, and the need for a local government.[13] But there was strong support for Hayes, whom the people considered one of their own, and reverence for her father's memory. Her scribbling visitors found no Force residents who'd speak against the doctor.

All three journalists seemed to have stepped inside the same miner's home. In unison, they contrasted the grimy exterior with the spotless inte-

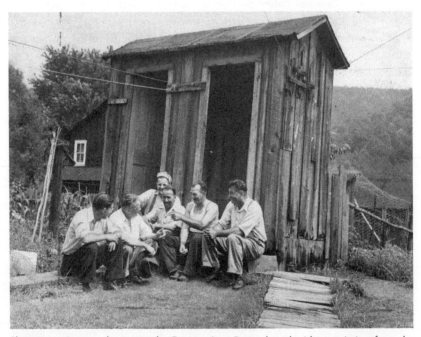

Shawmut miners gather around a Force privy. *Reproduced with permission from the Historical Society of Pennsylvania*

rior. Freshly painted and wallpapered, the kitchen sparkled with appliances bought and installed by its miner tenant. It might have been a model home, except for the missing faucets.

Judy Shepard of the *Post* slipped away from the group. Shepard, who would cowrite a guide to the young state of Israel, encouraging the avoidance of canned tours, interrupted a mailman on his rounds to ask him about Hayes. If she was probing the depth of support, she got her answer. "She's one swell kid," replied James Dorney, the postal worker. "I've known her for years. There are not more than half a dozen people in this whole valley who dislike her, and that half dozen are company officials."[14]

For the three women, as well as other journalists, Lambert continued to argue that Force, Byrnedale, and Hollywood had surpassed the typical coal town's twenty-five-year life, so it made no economic sense to modernize them. His reasoning was undermined by the miners' offer to contribute the labor and cover the costs.

But no matter. As one miner said in Shepard's piece—anonymously, probably because he feared for his job—"The owners just want to keep us down in the mud. They've had us down for forty years. That's why they won't let us improve this place."[15]

The trio interviewed Lambert as well, apparently by phone. Speaking to Kahn, he dropped a new bombshell: contradicting Campbell of the state health authority, who'd promised Shawmut's cooperation in decontaminating soil and wells, Lambert said Shawmut would do nothing while the strike was on and while Hayes was involved. "When the miners return to work, the company will sit down with the mine committee and discuss the doctor's demands. The men themselves do not favor all of them," said Lambert.[16] That last comment, as would become evident, had some truth to it. Lambert had found small fissures in Hayes's base to chip away at, through the snooping of private detective F. J. Erich.

Again, indoor bathrooms were a point of contention. Some miners didn't think powder rooms were worth striking about. At any rate, not every family crowded into a rented, boxlike house was willing or able to do remodeling. Speaking to the women reporters, Hayes stressed that she didn't insist on bathrooms. Still, in Kahn's widely read AP report, they resurged in a list of chief demands, along with a sewage system and running water.

Another threat to solidarity came from the UMWA's continued neutrality. Lambert falsely told a UP reporter that the miners had defied back-to-work orders to maintain their "outlaw strike." Representing the Force and Byrnedale locals, Ross Pentz countered that the UMWA had neither condemned nor condoned the walkout. It was a weak counterattack, but he had nothing else.

The eyes of the world were on Bennett's Valley. On August 2, the photos and features filed in Force ran in papers throughout the nation. Letters to Hayes came from servicemen who'd read about her in *Stars and Stripes*. In Force, Julia Shawell stayed an additional day. The *Philadelphia Record*, having already run her first piece about Force, had plans to showcase another.

Each of the three women who interviewed Hayes had something in common with her. Covering professional sports when women were barred from the press box, Kahn refused to be intimidated. Shepard spent the last chapter of her long life as a Washington, DC, community organizer, fighting for seniors' rights to home care. Yet it was Shawell, the former culture critic and gossip columnist, who made the strongest case for Hayes, vividly describing a day in the doctor's life and presenting the valley's pressing needs through facts and statistics.

Before agreeing to take Shawell on a ride-along, Hayes may have seen her previous day's piece about Force. Surely, she would have heard about it

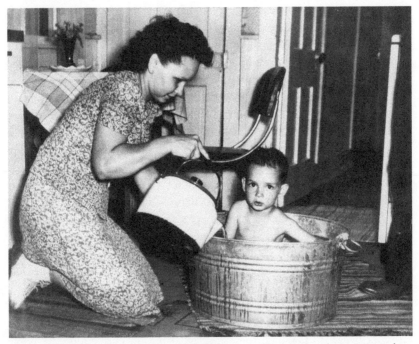

Force resident Jean Agosti bathes a little brother. *Reproduced with permission from the Historical Society of Pennsylvania*

from one of her Philadelphia-based siblings. To interest the *Record*'s readership, Shawell had written that Catherine and Vincent shared a practice in the city. For the same reason, she'd contacted Helen. Usually aloof from the family, Helen, like Catherine, had urged Shawell to go to Force and see conditions for herself.

So, here she was to see the doctor at work. For the first piece, Shawell had somehow cornered Lambert into praising Hayes's professional skills. "She's a good doctor, and the people in Force like her. In fact, she's well-liked in the whole territory. But she went on a tirade on this thing," Lambert had told the *Record*, most likely anticipating the warm reception that Shawell was bound to witness.[17]

If the journalist and the physician found time to chat, they would have discovered much in common. Like Hayes, Shawell was one of many siblings. She began her reporting career in early adulthood, commuting to New York from her comfortable home in Elizabeth, New Jersey. Before she was thirty, her engineer father died. Shawell's widowed mother took a low-paying job as a stenographer, while daughter Julia became the primary breadwinner.

A few years later, Shawell published a novel, *Autumn's Here*, about a "modern American family" in which a capable daughter is the sole supporter. Promotional copy for the book asked, "Should she break family ties, live only for Michael? Or must she forget the man whose love is the very essence of her existence?"

The book came out in 1937, the year Betty Hayes brought her hospital colleague, Rudolph Marburg, home to meet her family. Now he was married. So, too, was her former Penn State instructor LeRoy Voris, whose love, in romance-novel terms, had been the very essence of her existence until she found she must forget him. But she hadn't really done so.

Now, the two capable daughters of different families were bumping down village roads in Hayes's car. In her first piece, Shawell had presented this real-life tension between Dr. Hayes's modern medical and sanitary views and the age-old indifference of Force. Hayes's relatively recent medical training was also mentioned. As in her fictional portrayal of a new kind of American family, Shawell linked modernity to enlightenment.

Nevertheless, she was not above using some "age-old" techniques to paint a sympathetic portrait of a country doctor. In her long second feature, as Hayes slows before a patient's door, children jump on her car's running board, crying, "Dr. Betty!" Women shower Hayes with flowers and vegetables, weeping at the news of her imminent departure. A miner declares, "I wouldn't even take it if Dr. Betty didn't prescribe it." The *Record* also made clear that Hayes wouldn't be satisfied by the kind of cleanup and disinfection the state was proposing.[18]

It was a compelling narrative, anchored by nuts and bolts. Shawell managed to keep the story flowing while reporting the average rent in Force ($7.20) and the wages of the top-earning miners ($9 to $10 per hour, a record set in wartime). Included, too, were Hayes's prestrike monthly income ($40 directly from the company and $310 from the miners' payroll deductions) and the number of babies she'd delivered (142).

The next day, news from Force occupied almost an entire broadsheet page of the *Record*. Shawell's feature appeared under a montage of photos showing mining families coping with abominable conditions. Hayes's now-familiar headshot was also in the mix. Shawell had defied the misogynistic expectations of the paper's managing editor, Walter Lister. Interviewed about the new role of women in the wartime newsroom, he had replied, "Sloppiness is the one word that covers everything." He said that women journalists "write well enough," but "too many" fail to "ask the right questions," "don't get specific information," and "lack imagination."[19]

There was a sidebar, too: "Catholic Leader Cites Force, Pa., as Bad 'Example.'" The leader was Monsignor Luigi G. Ligutti, director of the Iowa-based National Catholic Rural Life Conference, dedicated to keeping rural Catholics on the land. He'd been speaking at a Philadelphia college when the *Record* asked him for comments about Force, which he'd learned of by reading the paper. A former "company priest," Ligutti was familiar with conditions in mining camps. As he spoke out, the bishop in Erie remained quiet about these events in his diocese.

In the same issue of the *Record* appeared the editorial, "An Indignant Physician Prescribes for Us All." Before the twenty-first century turned "angry woman" into a term of derision, the left-leaning Philadelphia paper congratulated Hayes for her rage. "Philadelphia has disgraceful slums for the same reason Force has contaminated wells—because too few people have been angry enough to fight to end these menaces to public health and community welfare," said the editorial. It added that the doctor had already obtained some results in that "the mining company is going to do 'something.'"[20]

But was that true? On the same day, the *Pittsburgh Press*'s editorial board also praised "plucky" Hayes, but more cautiously. "Scarcely anyone approves of coal miners striking in these days when their product is so vital to prosecution of the war," said the editorial, but in this case, the miners have been "reasonable," agreeing to go back to work as soon as the company made a move toward improvements. Bill Agosti was quoted as saying,

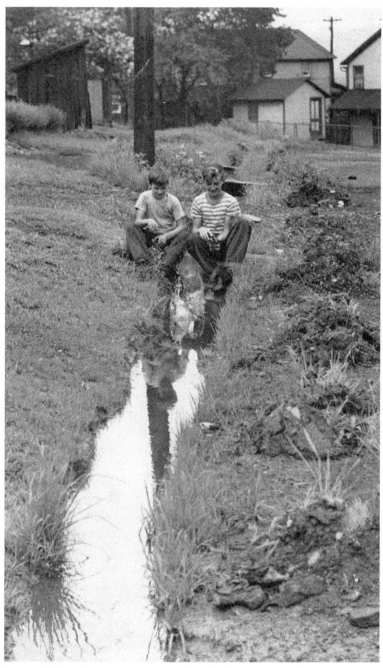

Force children play near a sewage-filled ditch. *Reproduced with permission from the Historical Society of Pennsylvania*

"We just want them to say they'll do something." The editorial concluded, "If the company won't 'do something' on its own initiative, the State Health Department undoubtedly will order action."[21] That hadn't happened yet. Indeed, the state had still not finished its survey of water quality.

In the same edition, the *Press* ran a news story filed from DuBois. Lambert's latest comment: "We haven't agreed to anything, and the State has made no demands on us." He also revealed his progress on a divide-and-conquer strategy. Admitting to the local reporter that the coal in Force's Proctor No. 1 mine might be worked for "six or seven more years," he also had to acknowledge that Proctor No. 2, opened two decades later, could potentially be worked longer than that. "But it is at Force where all the trouble is," said Lambert. His hired snoop was earning his keep.[22]

The DuBois newspaper had also detected some fault lines, or so it said. A "water system" was not demanded by "the men," wrote the *Courier-Express*, thus excluding Hayes without naming sources, but "they do demand the removal of contamination from the water in the wells." For these unidentified males, "Water and sewage systems are things for consideration in a longer program," presumably after the strike was called off.[23] The paper added that it "understood" that the state health agency had nearly completed its water survey, with any action required of the company soon to be announced. Virtually a mouthpiece for Shawmut, on these matters, its reporting was reliable.

That piece ran on a Saturday. It was the end of a week in which Hayes, mentioned in miles of lines of print, was said to be "surprised at the furor she has aroused." She also resented the intrusion on her privacy. Profiling Hayes for the *Pittsburgh Press*'s Sunday edition, the paper's DuBois contributor wrote, "As for romance in her own life, she brushes off all questions about it. 'Leave that out of it,' she laughed. That has nothing to do with it."[24]

Laughter yielded to bad temper as the unfortunate *Press* stringer asked Hayes to comment on a popular book that had been adapted to film, A. J. Cronin's *The Citadel*. Based on the author's medical career in Welsh mining country, the plot involves a typhoid outbreak caused by sewage leaking into wells. When local authorities fail to respond, a concerned physician blows up the sewer that's at fault, forcing the construction of a new one. The story casts the doctor's actions in a heroic light.

Despite the striking parallels between her situation and this well-known work, Hayes seemed to resent the question. "I didn't have to read a book to get my ideas for this campaign," she snapped. "I got them by just looking at things here in the village." Struggling to remain charitable, the reporter wrote, "She has a ready smile, but her face can become grim and determined when she talks about her fight."[25]

But of all that had been printed, six spare lines threatened to change the game. They began, "Wanted—Mine Physician" and concluded with the address of F. D. Lambert. Shawmut had placed its first ad in the *Journal of the American Medical Association.*

The next week began with President Truman's announcement that the world's first atomic bomb had been dropped on the Japanese city of Hiroshima. On that same Monday, Hayes unleashed a weapon of her own. She left town without announcing her destination. The miners postponed a community meeting set for Wednesday. No one seemed to know if Hayes would be back by then.

Even one day with no doctor within reach could be consequential. In the two days that elapsed between Hayes's resignation and the start of the strike, a miner had injured his hand and waited over three hours to be taken to St. Marys Hospital. With no pharmacy in the valley, Hayes was also the only source of medications. Nevertheless, she went.

It was a "vacation," she later told the press, but that seems disingenuous. Had it been planned, the miners wouldn't have scheduled a meeting for Thursday. More likely, she was testing the resolve of her allies. In league with the company, the state was poised to propose a quick fix to a grave problem, and some men seemed eager to settle for it.

Hayes had warned them: they had to line up solidly behind her, or she'd take her bag and leave. By the evening of that historic day, she was dining with friends in Kingston. Years before, she'd lived and worked quietly near Nesbitt Memorial Hospital, where she'd done her residency. Now a Wilkes-Barre paper, the *Times-Leader*, was watching her every move. Within hours, the paper reported that Hayes was the guest of Charles L. Shafer, a prominent physician associated with Nesbitt, and his wife, Mary.[26] On this particular day, there would have been plenty to talk about: a son of the Shafers was serving in the Pacific. The couple also might have been interested in Hayes's future plans. Did she plan to resume her private practice near Nesbitt someday? According to another Wilkes-Barre paper, the *Recorder*, her Kingston friends had expected her back after one year in Newfoundland.[27] Then came her father's death and the detour to Force.

Besides putting any wavering strikers on notice, Hayes could have had emotional reasons for her impromptu visit. Her mother was all packed and ready to move. Facing formidable adversaries and dealing with sudden celebrity, Hayes may have turned to Dr. Shafer, sixty-two, in search of a father figure.

It's also possible that the classified ad in the American Medical Association's journal had prompted the visit. Ads for mining-town physicians were not unusual in the publication's widely read classified section, but some specified licensing requirements. Just inches below Shawmut's ad was one that began, "Wanted—for mine practice by September 15; West Virginia license or reciprocate; under 55 years; sober." By contrast, the ad seeking a replacement for Hayes said nothing about a Pennsylvania license or eligibility for it. Nor was there an upper age limit, which was then legal, or any mention of sobriety.

Shafer was on the State Board of Medical Education and Licensure. Hayes might have wanted his assurance that any unlicensed suitors for her job would invite the board's scrutiny. Shafer might also have been involved in granting reciprocity to applicants licensed in other states. Three years before, the company had tried to block Hayes from taking her job—preferring, in her words, an "unlicensed quack." She might have sought Shafer's help in deterring Shawmut's attempts to try that again.

There were sure to be applicants. The ad had overstated the "outside revenues" that could be expected beyond the small base salary and the miners' contributions. To be sure, Hayes's normal caseload included patients unconnected with Shawmut. According to the ad, additional billings would total $300 monthly (equivalent to $4,300 in 2020) over payroll. Journalists didn't ask Hayes about her outside income, but another Pennsylvania country doctor wrote a column in praise of Hayes, noting that conditions must be very bad indeed to make a physician quit a "lucrative" mine practice. That writer, however, had no personal knowledge of Hayes or her income, which hadn't tempted her siblings to trade places with her. Considering the hardships in the area, the difficulties of bill collection, and Shawmut's other falsehoods, the advertised figure was probably vastly overblown.

Still, as Hayes knew, it was bound to draw responses and, even with the strike on, the miners had to find a way to involve her in screening candidates. After two nights in Kingston, she headed back to Force, reappearing as suddenly as she'd gone. She'd left on the day that Hiroshima was destroyed, returning as bombs fell on Nagasaki.

The end of the war was imminent, but most doctors would remain in the service for months. Those discharged weren't likely to seek postwar jobs in the nation's filthy coal towns, described by an admiral as worse than battle areas. Only desperate or unqualified practitioners were likely to apply.

There was another reason that Hayes wanted to be involved in the selection of a doctor. In theory, she was willing to step aside for a suitable replacement. In reality, she and her supporters weren't serious about the search. To the press and the state Unemployment Compensation Bureau, the miners said they were striking until "a doctor" was on the job. For the leaders, though, only a doctor with the last name of Hayes would do. Accepting her leadership and scientific guidance, they would see things through to a satisfactory conclusion.

Hayes returned to find that the state had finally posted boil-water notices on the well pumps. In screaming capital letters they began: DANGEROUS! DO NOT DRINK THE WATER and continued with the orders to boil. In her absence, the state had reported findings of sewage contamination in eleven of the twenty-one wells included in its survey.

The lab results scored points for the doctor and the strikers in press reports. Here was data—collected by a state authority, not a private lab—to support anecdotal complaints of misery and filth. However, boiling instructions were nothing more than what Hayes, and her father before her, had recommended for years. Moreover, by signaling that nearly half the wells were safe, the state was undermining her advice. There were high levels of iron and sulfur in those wells, making their water unpotable as well.

The real danger would come in the next steps. After releasing the water survey results, Campbell had dispatched a division chief to meet with Shawmut. Now that Hayes was the darling of the editorial pages, Harrisburg could no longer ignore her. James C. Bell, the head of the state health department's Division of Environmental Hygiene, agreed to meet with the "crusading" doctor. She still had no official role in the matter, but now millions of newspaper readers followed her every move.

Meanwhile, the descriptions of conditions in Force were subverting a public-relations campaign financed by the coal industry. Disastrous mine explosions and accidents weren't uncommon, and many Americans worried about the dangers faced by miners, as well as their wages and living conditions. To counter these concerns, while also addressing doubts about coal dependence, coal operators formed the National Bituminous Institute. Based in New York, the so-called institute worked with a Madison Avenue agency on magazine advertisements designed to burnish the industry's image.

One such ad included a question: a garage mechanic in Nashville asked, "What kind of homes do miners live in today?" In response, the institute wrote,

> For the most part, miners live in homes as attractive and comfortable as any other well-paid workers. Washing machines, radios, refrigerators, and other home appliances are commonly found in miners' homes. . . .
> When a miner lives in a company home, it is because he wants to.

Today company homes on company property are usually better than the average home in the sections where they are located.

A year after that ad ran in *Newsweek*, the *Atlantic*, and the *Saturday Evening Post*, the public learned there might be radios in those homes, but no toilets or running water. As publicity surrounded Force's filth, the institute's director tried to redirect attention to a model coal town under construction in Kentucky. However, it was impossible to divert the public eye from a physician described in one column as "the blond bombshell who is acting in the best traditions of the profession."[28] Shawmut was an industrial embarrassment.

When it came to state law, though, the tables were turned. Meeting with Bell, Hayes learned that the health department couldn't order Shawmut to do anything but make minor repairs to the wells and chlorinate the water. Hayes and Pentz came to accept this. Both criticized "loopholes" in state health laws, but they didn't take the matter to court.

Newly aware that state health laws could provide no help, Hayes addressed the first meeting open to "community representatives" from Force, Byrnedale, and Hollywood. It's unclear what that term meant. Coverage of the event suggests that the gathering exceeded the size of the usual miners' committee meeting. Rank-and-file members seemed to have attended, but it's unclear if their wives were there. Hayes might have been the only woman present. If other prominent valley residents were there—clergymen, independent grocers, or the Force Hotel proprietor—they weren't named.

The main item on the agenda had been announced in advance. Attendees approved a letter that invited company officials to another meeting scheduled a week hence, where the company and community could work out their "proportionate obligations" for sharing the cost and work of a real cleanup. Certified letters would be sent to Dickson at his New York refuge and to McBride and Lambert in St. Marys. Hayes called them invitations to a "showdown."

It wasn't the first challenge she had issued to the three executives. When Lambert had suggested that the miners' housing was a great deal for low rents, Hayes's retort delighted reporters. "Why don't the mine officials live here?" she'd said. Certified mail had more gravity than wisecracks. But she probably didn't expect any more of a response now than she had then.

Nonetheless, the invitation to a showdown—or "ultimatum," as the doctor also called it—supplied a hook for reporters covering the meeting, where Hayes denounced the toothless state health laws. She added that boil-water notices should have been posted on ten additional pumps. Not finding sewage contamination there, the health authority had left them alone. But Hayes said the water from those pumps, too, was "not potable" due to dangerous levels of iron and sulfur. She may have seen the results from the state water survey.

The other business discussed was less dramatic, but arguably more significant. A seven-member citizens' committee was formed to continue to press demands, with Hayes appointed to it. For the press, the formation of the citizens' committee—later called the community league or community committee—signaled that the protest in Force was more than a labor–management dispute. Other committee members were miners, including Bill Agosti, Joseph Shadick, and Tony Coccimiglio, president of the Force and Byrnedale locals. Perhaps its most important function was to include Hayes and give her a role other than "former company doctor."

Indeed, the company-doctor system was another item under discussion. The miners' attorney, Pentz, said commercial insurance would serve them better than Shawmut's medical plan. "I don't know of any but mining companies that elect to self-insure," he said, noting that only management benefited, taking a 10 percent administrative fee.[29]

In the meantime, though, many would-be company doctors were responding to the Shawmut ad, and the clock was ticking. The War Manpower Commission, the Unemployment Compensation Bureau, and the Solid Fuels Administration would all rule soon on whether the men were justified in leaving their jobs. The miners' claims hinged on the absence of a doctor. Even with her friend, Dr. Shafer, overseeing the licensing board, there was still some risk that a qualified applicant might turn up.

Defeated by the state, Hayes sought help at the federal level. U.S. Representative Leon Gavin spent an afternoon in Force, meeting with Hayes and touring the sights, which he described as "revolting" and "deplorable." "If conditions are no different in other mining communities than they are in Force, it might be well to examine, carefully analyze, and correct them throughout the state," said the congressman. Urging Shawmut officials to attend the upcoming meeting, he promised to monitor the situation and, if necessary, enlist the aid of his fellow Republican, Governor Martin. The lawmaker could do nothing more. The federal government, he said, had neither the authority nor obligation to make improvements.[30]

With the nation awaiting the announcement of peace—rumors had already sparked premature celebrations—reports of Gavin's meeting with "pretty Dr. Hayes" receded to the back pages of the papers. A Pulitzer Prize–winning reporter from the *Pittsburgh Post-Gazette*, Ray Sprigle had belatedly joined the ranks of those covering the story. Known for his

Stetson hat and corncob pipe, the fifty-eight-year-old made an unusual sight in Bennett's Valley, where he spent two days chatting up the residents in Force, Hollywood, and Byrnedale. He shared the local enthusiasm for firearms, and he was doubtless the first reporter they had met who'd once worked in a coal mine, just for a week, to get a story.

In Force, he joined some miners watching five men build a wooden form around the head of a well. The miners, skilled in carpentry, laughed at the time this was taking and the number of builders involved. The plan, approved by the state, was to pour concrete into the form. Speaking from Harrisburg, Campbell said other wells would be "protected" from contamination in this way, with no need for a sewage system. Hayes refused to be placated. "We're past halfway measures," she said.[31]

Declaring that its work was nearing completion, the state updated the results of its water survey. Not only were most of Force's wells contaminated, but so was one of its springs, the source of water for the homes in its silk-stocking district. When she'd invited the company executives to move to Force, Hayes had said, "I know just under what conditions those miners live, for I live among them myself."[32] Those words were truer than she'd suspected.

However, her indoor bathrooms spared her from a fresh humiliation. Emboldened by its recent victory in state health matters, Shawmut informed its tenants that it would no longer clean out their outhouses. In a letter, Lambert pointed to a provision of the housing lease requiring tenants to keep their premises "neat and clean." That provision, the tenants were informed, included the privies.[33]

Evidently, this meant the end of services provided by the "honey dipper," or sewage-removal service, which was routinely provided by mining companies. The system was far from ideal. A miner living in another company-owned town, Kenivir, Kentucky, described its inadequacies:

> The coal company has a wagon that starts at the uppermost [*sic*] part of this large mining camp and dips this waste out of each toilet until the wagon is full, and by the time it reaches the dump, which is some two or three hundred feet from our houses, the contents of the wagon is [*sic*] scattered all over the mining camp running all over the road and down in front of the houses.[34]

Pennsylvania state law required the use of covered vehicles for this purpose, but none were available in Force. Speaking to the press about the company's refusal to do waste removal, Pentz said, "For forty years, the company has always done that when it was done at all."[35]

As Lambert had said of the strike, "We'll have to see who gets tired [of] waiting first." Determined to wear down its opponents, Shawmut had embarked on a campaign of harassment. The Kentucky miner who gave the graphic description of toilet-dipping also described its absence: "In some of these toilets waste is stacked up one to two feet above the seat." The already intolerable conditions in Bennett's Valley had suddenly worsened.

Shawmut's next punitive move was more targeted, aimed directly at the strike leaders. The company withdrew the occupational deferments of eleven men, who promptly received draft notices. Responding to press questions, Lambert said, "We don't see why these men's names shouldn't be given to the draft board when they are loafing around and trying to get unemployment compensation while they are on strike." The reclassified men were scheduled for pre-induction medical exams in Harrisburg, one day before the scheduled showdown meeting.[36]

"Perfect timing," quipped Hayes, pointing out that one of the induct-ees was on the miners' committee, another was a brother of its chairman, while a third was a member's son. She also noted that the Truman admin-istration was asking the armed forces to release miners from military service. In the same week that the Force men got their notices, the director of war mobilization advised draft boards everywhere to give miners deferments. A severe coal shortage was anticipated, and more diggers were needed.

One Force resident was immediately suspected of complicity. Walter Mowrey, a bookkeeper for Shawmut, served on the three-man draft board. The board chairman strenuously insisted that Mowrey had no role in se-lecting the miners because rules prohibited him from doing so. But it's no wonder that the affair raised questions. Many believed it bore the finger-prints of another one-time company bookkeeper: Peter McBride.

Significantly, Lambert didn't release the names of any Hollywood miners. As residents of Clearfield County registered with the DuBois draft board, those men eluded McBride's grip. At any rate, the company had other reasons for sparing the men of the Hollywood local. They were more ambivalent about the strike.

Less than forty-eight hours before the miners headed for the Har-risburg induction center, Truman announced Japan's unconditional sur-render. In DuBois, people ran out of movie theaters where seven o'clock showings had just begun, joining the noisy crowds gathering on the streets. Motorists leaned on their horns and formed traffic jams as office workers abandoned their dinner tables to run back to their offices and throw ticker tape and ripped paper from the windows.

In its own version of the iconic Times Square photo, the *Courier-Express* described a soldier kissing his sweetheart under the traffic light at Long Avenue and Brady Street. The paper also noted that behind the joyous shouting were the tears of the relatives of "nearly one hundred of the city's finest young men who made the supreme sacrifice."[37] Noisemakers and firecrackers were heard until 1:00 a.m. when rain soaked the revelers and the homemade confetti.

On August 15, V-J Day, the employees of Shawmut Mining had another reason to celebrate. All wartime employment restrictions were lifted. The miners were released from their jobs, free to work anywhere. On that same day, the DuBois paper wrote that the Solid Fuels Administration would not intervene in the strike. "We can't very well order the men back to work without a doctor," said a district director.[38]

Still, these were small gains compared to the company's recent display of political muscle. With the announced showdown scheduled two days hence, no response had come from Shawmut Mining. As Hayes and the strikers celebrated the Allied victory, they must have felt the need for a new strategy.

For the miners who had received induction notices, there was better news. The Truman administration announced that men over the age of twenty-six would no longer be subject to the draft. Only one man in the group was eligible for service. Nevertheless, McBride probably thought the exercise worthwhile. His message had gotten through: activism would be punished. Conversely—or so the Hollywood miners may have understood—cooperation would be rewarded.

The so-called showdown meeting was a bust. Probably surprising no one, the Shawmut officials failed to materialize at the meeting place, Ross Pentz's DuBois law office. Some reporters were on hand. Other than that, only the miners' committee attended, along with Hayes and Pentz. It was Friday afternoon, the start of the first postwar weekend, but the mood wasn't celebratory. Suddenly freed to work anywhere—although only a few had requested releases—the miners weren't sure of their next move.

Pentz spoke of the possibility of forming a housing authority that could finance improvements. Or the three villages might incorporate as boroughs and pass ordinances requiring Shawmut to clean up. Besides the time involved, both avenues would require substantial contributions from the company, and the protest leaders were beginning to believe Shawmut's cries of poverty. Doubts were settling over the valley.

When the first reports of the strike broke, Lambert had told Elaine Kahn of the Associated Press, "A railroad which is in receivership owns the capital stock of our company, so the Federal Court of Western Pennsylvania has jurisdiction over and operates the properties."[39] On Dickson's Shawmut Mining letterhead, he was the company president; however, he was also the receiver of the PS&N and its mining subsidiaries. McBride was the assistant receiver.

Those titles had recently taken on new meaning. It was no secret in financial circles that Shawmut was in receivership, a form of bankruptcy. The average person hadn't paid much attention until the *Pittsburgh Press* took a fresh look at the company in light of Hayes's demands. A week before V-J day, an investigative report in the paper concluded that Shawmut was "broke" and "can't afford to make those improvements."[40]

The rest of the piece gave a brief history of "one of the most amazing receiverships in the entire country," which seemed to be the longest on record, having started forty years before. Dickson, appointed receiver in 1923, had managed to increase the company's indebtedness by millions of dollars. In a refinancing scheme approved by a federal court, he'd issued receiver's certificates for $2,044,350 bearing 6 percent interest. No interest been paid since then, and no certificates had been retired. Hence, the company owed more than $3 million to certificate holders.

Dickson was contacted by phone and given ample chance to respond. He had an answer for everything. A 1942 lawsuit filed by two unhappy certificate holders had been put on hold because of the war. At any rate, the two represented less than 1 percent of the certificate holders, not a truly representative group with which he might negotiate. They were demanding a reorganization plan, which Dickson had tried to file long before, only to be told it was "premature" because the Great Depression was on then. Regarding the certificate holders' complaint that they never received any financial reports, Dickson agreed but noted that "it was not required."[41]

The page 2 article was dense reading, although a line above the humdrum headline popped out. "Shawmut's Broke—But Flat," it said, while a subhead declared that the company "Has Been in Hock to Creditors Since 1905." A capsule form of the piece ran in the *Press*'s Letter-from-the-Hometown section, a weekly digest of news designed for mailing to service members. The column presented the news as an update for overseas readers already familiar with the "dramatic fight for health" in Force.

But would it be fight or flight? A third option, discussed in Pentz's office, was for everyone to pack up collectively and seek jobs elsewhere. Another meeting was set for the following week. It would be held at the Force church hall, with the miners' wives urged to attend. A vote would be taken on whether to abandon the three towns to their mud and filth. The strikers called it mass migration.

Speaking to the press, Hayes framed this as a brash ultimatum. "Now it's all or nothing with us. Either we are going to live like human beings, or we're going to get out. All of us."[42] But the suggestion had probably originated with the practical Pentz, who could see no other path forward, and behind the doctor's bold words was a sense of desperation.

As reported by the *Courier-Express*, revelations of the company's "weakened financial situation" had shaken the resolve of Hayes and the mining committee. Reporting on a meeting of the strike leaders held at Pentz's office, the paper stated, "In the end, they concluded it was practically useless to fight the situation . . . and that the smart thing to do would be to get out." As the DuBois paper saw it, the sole purpose of the next community meeting would be to present the "recommendations for mass emigration."[43]

With privies growing filthier by the day, state-approved chlorinated water, and a cash-poor yet politically powerful landlord, the communities had reached a low point. The idea of convincing every household in each town to move *en masse* seemed daunting, if not preposterous, but it sounded more militant than surrender.

As it happened, there was no need to worry. The *Pittsburgh Post-Gazette* had just printed the first installment of Ray Sprigle's series about Force under the banner "Plague Spots," and Shawmut officials were frantically trying to make it disappear.

In St. Marys, where the rafts of white-collar workers employed by Shawmut had suddenly stopped getting paid, not a copy of the *Post-Gazette* could be found for purchase. The protesters in Bennett's Valley had an influential new friend.

5

CRACKS AND PATCHES

If ace reporter Ray Sprigle hadn't entered the picture, the miners would have settled. At least that's how Dickson saw it. Millions of words supporting Hayes had already been printed around the world. But nothing provoked the company like the three-part series by the veteran *Pittsburgh Post-Gazette* staff writer. Dickson was so incensed that he forbade Shawmut employees from ever talking to the press again.

Just as everyone was beginning to accept the company's excuses, Sprigle punched a hole in them.

Later, a St. Marys grocer used a worn typewriter ribbon and loose-leaf paper to tap out copies of Sprigle's lengthy pieces before returning the originals to their owner. The *Post-Gazette* had been suppressed from news-stands in St. Marys, the grocer noted, as he passed along his clandestine transcript. But outside that snug borough, Sprigle's series was widely read, reaching into the White House. It elevated a human-interest story into an exposé of the abuse of bankruptcy laws.

Much of this had to do with Sprigle's status at the *Post-Gazette*, where he'd been the city editor before choosing to return to reporting. He had a loyal readership, the support of his publisher, and the resources for in-depth reports. He won his 1938 Pulitzer for producing documents proving that U.S. Supreme Court Justice Hugo Black had once belonged to the Ku Klux Klan. But Sprigle was also known for assuming disguises and false identities to go undercover. For an investigation of a city hospital serving as a homeless shelter, he'd become the derelict "Ed Crawford."

More recently, he'd posed as the black-market butcher "Alois Vondich" to spotlight the government's failure to enforce price controls and wartime food rationing. His articles produced arrests and sparked a Senate investigation. They also cost the paper $2,000 in meat and truck rental fees. Sprigle's "Plague Spots" series about the noxious towns in Bennett's Valley cost less, but consumed time. Unlike the women journalists who had laid the groundwork in Force, he could write with a free hand. Measuring five feet, ten inches, with his signature Stetson hat and corncob pipe, Ray Sprigle stood no danger of being branded a sob sister.

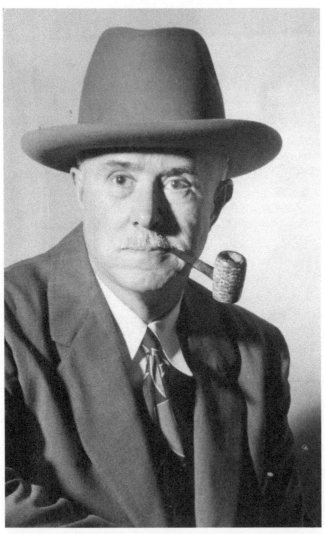

Pittsburgh Post-Gazette reporter Ray Sprigle. *Ray Sprigle Papers and Photographs, Detre Library & Archives, Heinz History Center*

The first installment of his series on Shawmut's coal towns contained little new information, but having spent two days in them, Sprigle introduced rankings. "Force is the filthiest . . . Byrnedale is almost as bad. Hollywood is just an ordinary unkempt industrial slum." Adding to the praise already heaped on Hayes, he described her as a "110-pound medical whirlwind," a "full-fledged insurrecto," and "leader of a resistance movement" that was "long overdue."[1]

But it was the second installment that Dickson had dreaded most. Here, Sprigle explained why Shawmut's "flat broke" status had been its normal operating mode for nearly half a century, never standing in the way of executive salaries. Like Chester Potter of the *Pittsburgh Press*, Sprigle noted that the company's issuance of receiver's certificates had augmented its debts. But by presenting the mounting liabilities as part of a long-standing financial scheme, Sprigle demolished the company's defense. He wrote,

> Operation under a receivership simplifies or eliminates entirely many of the problems that beset ordinary business . . . Shawmut is always broke. And that provides a ready excuse for anything and everything that is put up to the receiver in the way of suggestions for improvements. . . . But Shawmut still pays the salaries of Receiver Dickson and Assistant Receiver McBride.[2]

Contrary to what Dickson had told the *Press* about his lack of filing obligations, Sprigle found court documents that explicitly required financial reports from the receiver. Yet for two decades, Dickson had filed "not one scrap of paper" to indicate where the company's money was going, including the salary he paid himself.

Nevertheless, Sprigle had located a figure that proved accurate. Dickson was pulling down $15,000 a year, far more than the monthly $250 reported in the *Press*. Despite rolling up deficits during every year of his receivership, sometimes in the hundreds of thousands, "Attorney Dickson has drawn down from the wrecked and insolvent string of companies more than a quarter of a million dollars—to be specific $240,000—at the rate of $15,000 a year," Sprigle wrote. Although unable to provide the assistant receiver's salary, he noted, "Mr. McBride isn't having any privy or sewage problem" in his "very, very nice" brick "mansion" in St. Marys.[3] Side-by-side photos of the McBride home and a miner's shack accompanied the piece.

There were no quotes from the receiver or assistant receiver, who'd thrown Sprigle out of their respective offices. McBride's menacing appearance had enabled him to clear his St. Marys quarters "with no argument from the inquiring reporter," Sprigle wrote. Traveling across the state line to Wellsville, he reported that "Receiver Dickson was extremely courteous and pleasant" but begged "to be excused" from answering questions in the "pious hope that everyone would just keep quiet and all this hullaballoo would just lie down and quietly die."[4]

The third installment of the series addressed Shawmut's laments about its obligations to provide worker housing. Sprigle compared rents and tax assessments to prove that the company was "making a pretty good thing out of its sewage-soaked shacks." Other than that, he covered much of the ground already traversed. Sanitizing the mining families for white, native-born, middle-class readers, he described the "third-generation" children as "well behaved," with the girls "unbelievably clean in stiffly starched dresses."[5] Over the years, he told readers, many had left to become professionals, including forty nurses, three engineers, and dozens of teachers.

Attending a committee meeting in Hayes's living room—where he'd become something of a fixture—Sprigle asked the miners why they continued to live in squalor when they could probably get jobs elsewhere. Bill Agosti replied, "We don't like it outside. [We're] just mountain people at heart, I guess." Curating and arranging quotes for dramatic effect, Sprigle used as Agosti's closing remark, "What I don't see is why we shouldn't be able to live decently here as well as anywhere else."[6]

Hayes and her proponents—Ray Sprigle now among them—hoped the women of the community would attend the public meeting. In that spirit, Sprigle ended his series with an apt quote from miner Joseph Shadick: "I wonder how many women died long before their time because they had to struggle day after day with these man-killing pumps."[7]

Two days after that remark appeared in print, a young Force woman died, not from pumping water, but by suicide. Lena DePaoli, twenty-six, used a high-powered rifle to shoot herself in the spleen while other household members were out for the evening. They returned to find her dying but conscious. They attempted to summon Hayes, who was out on a house call and couldn't be contacted. The phone service cut off at night.

The young woman was finally brought to a DuBois hospital at around 11:00 p.m., only to be pronounced dead within minutes of arrival. According to the death certificate, she'd survived for four hours. When conscious, she'd expressed "no remorse," the *Courier-Express* reported, also noting that authorities could find "no connection between the tragedy and the sanitation troubles of the Force community."[8]

But Hayes did, stating publicly and to the press, "She just grew so tragically tired of living in Force that death seemed the easy way out. This is not a good life we live here," said Hayes, adding that there'd been "no love affair."[9] The doctor and the dead woman had lived close to one another, both single women, perhaps knowing each other well. Or Hayes could have been speaking as a physician to quash rumors of a pregnancy. If the family of the deceased woman had any objections, they didn't make them known.

As DePaoli's body lay on view at her parents' home, the community meeting convened in the church hall. Wives who attended were seated apart from their husbands in the front row, where an AP photographer could easily get them into a picture. The event began with a report by Hayes about letters she'd received from "our boys overseas." She said some wouldn't return to Bennett's Valley because "they can see no reason for fighting for something on foreign soil and then not even having it in their own homes."[10]

Mass migration was no longer under serious discussion. Much had changed since the appearance of Sprigle's *Post-Gazette* series. Shawmut's newsstand blockade hadn't succeeded outside of St. Marys. The wire services and papers everywhere were reporting Dickson's $15,000 salary, along with the newer report that McBride was pulling down $12,000 (a figure later found to be somewhat inflated, although Dickson's was accurate). The flat-broke company and its record-breaking receivership were raising a lot of questions.

Invoking Lena De Paoli's memory, Hayes and the union leaders urged the community to fight on, a daunting prospect for many. A decision from the state unemployment bureau was expected soon, but even if it went in the miners' favor, the five-week penalty meant their missed paychecks were gone forever. Some families had other income; DePaoli, for one, had been employed at a St. Marys carbon plant. For others, debts were mounting at the valley's three independent grocery stores.

Turning to other business, the miners authorized Hayes to approve or reject applications from physicians seeking to replace her. Moreover, final candidates would have to present themselves in person for an interview. Of eighteen applications received, the company had referred two to the miners. The men had declined to approve them, stating they didn't know enough about the candidates' qualifications. There were questions from some attendees about Hayes's commitment to staying on, perhaps prompted by her mother's move. As would later become apparent, not everyone saw her as irreplaceable.

The townspeople needed a project to paper over their differences, and the media needed news. Feeding both needs, Ray Sprigle raised his hand and was recognized. He moved that telegrams be sent to UMWA President

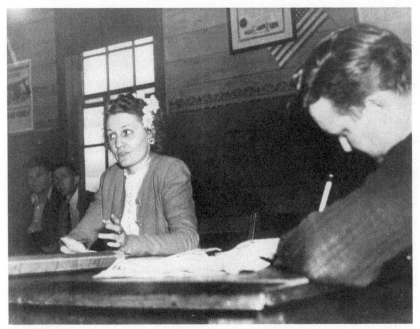

Dr. Betty Hayes addresses the community meeting. *Reproduced with permission from the Historical Society of Pennsylvania*

John L. Lewis and Pennsylvania Governor Edward Martin asking for their support. The motion was seconded and passed without objection. The text of the telegrams was given to reporters. They cried out for help "in the name of humanity." Obviously taking a hand in the writing, Sprigle had composed the next day's headlines.

By modern journalistic standards, Sprigle had violated the rule prohibiting reporters from becoming part of the story. But of all the news outlets present, only the *Pittsburgh Press* found his participation in the meeting worth mentioning.

Other business at the meeting sought to widen the scope of the struggle. Thus far, a Shawmut mine had stayed open in Brandy Camp, northwest of the three striking towns. A decision was made to urge the Brandy Camp miners to join the strike. Sprigle probably played a role in this. His "Plague Spots" series made several mentions of Brandy Camp, describing it as "the most dilapidated" of the Shawmut-owned coal communities and "at least a runner-up" to Force in terms of filth. With that decision, "the little people of Force, sitting on the hard benches of St. Joseph's Church hall," ended their meeting, Sprigle wrote.[11] The telegrams went out early the next day from the Western Union office in DuBois.

John L. Lewis joined the disappearing act. Seeking comment from him after news of the telegram broke, the United Press found him unavailable. A union spokesman attempted to deflect attention from Force, referring the UP reporter to a recent *United Mine Workers Journal* editorial warning coal operators to upgrade their housing or face labor shortages. The editorial observed that veterans were shunning the coalfields, and brides "want nothing of coal camp life." In the same issue was the journal's first news piece about Hayes and the work stoppage. A rehash of items printed elsewhere, the report was out of date by the time it appeared.

The UMWA's response to the telegram was ambiguous at best. "We are unable to have a revision of the contract on this issue, as you suggest," said the reply, noting that a measure designed to eliminate "such unbearable conditions" had failed during negotiations of the last contract. The only encouragement, if it could be interpreted as such, came in the final sentence, which began, "Assuredly your Union will do everything possible to help remedy the situation," while concluding with the puzzling phrase, "but we cannot compel action by force."[12] The response was signed by John J. Mattes, an international board member, who wrote that Lewis was temporarily absent from the office. Lewis, who routinely answered letters from his members about small matters, kept his distance from the high-profile events in Force, at least publicly.

But behind the scenes, Lewis was taking note of the sanitation struggle and his district president's response to it. Within days of his "temporary absence," he was back at his desk, handling correspondence from other Pennsylvania locals urging the UMWA to take a stand. The suggested wave of sympathy strikes hadn't materialized, but miners were taking up their pens.

Some pointed fingers at James Mark. "Is it possible that a fight for better Sanitation . . . is not in favor with Dist. #2 president?" asked the officers of a local in Dagus Mines, Pennsylvania. "He has not contacted the Force Miners. Neither has he made any effort to settle this dispute." Lewis replied, promising to "continue to give every consideration possible" to "conditions in Force."[13] His signature on that message is perhaps the only surviving evidence of his awareness of the struggle there. Responding a few days later to a similar letter from a local in Roscoe, Pa., he advised them to take up the matter with District 2 officials instead. Mark, who customarily sought Lewis's guidance on dealing with unauthorized strikes, seems to have been left to his own devices.

Lewis's abandonment of the issue went mostly unnoticed. A *Post-Gazette* piece, not bylined but obviously written by Sprigle, spoke of "indications" that the union was about to give "its powerful backing" to the struggle.[14] The only loud criticism of Lewis came from the *Daily Worker*, published by the Communist Party USA. The party had been highly critical of the UMWA president for calling wartime strikes while the Soviet Union was battling Hitler. Now, its paper excoriated "the Great John L" for leaving Force to twist in the wind. "His face must have been red lately at the unexpected publicity from coast to coast given to conditions existing in American mine towns," wrote Elizabeth Gurley Flynn, and "by a woman at that." A well-known feminist and activist, Flynn wrote columns lauding Hayes for "blowing the lid" off a situation that, in her view, Lewis had tolerated for far too long.[15]

Hunting for miners similarly critical of Lewis, the *Daily Worker*'s Philadelphia editor, Walter Lowenfels, hitched a truck ride to Force with a photographer. They received a lukewarm reception from Hayes and the coal diggers. Dependent on the union for disability and other benefits, they had to be "damn careful" about what they said, as one miner put it. Bill Agosti commented that housing and sanitation should have been negotiated at national conventions. Then he dropped the subject. As for Hayes, with the Cold War taking shape, she seemed less than enthused about this visitor. She chatted with him but wouldn't allow herself to be photographed, suggesting shots of sewage instead because "that's the story." Nevertheless, Lowenfels—who'd written poetry in Paris before devoting himself to leftist journalism—was smitten. Describing her as "Norse-like" and "moderately tall," he seems to have confused her heroic dimensions with her physical ones. He compared her to Ulysses S. Grant, determined to take Richmond no matter how long it took.[16]

Now that the telegram had been sent to UMWA headquarters, James Mark was tracked down for comment. It was widely known that the District 2 president had no real autonomy. A resident of DuBois, Mark was corralled into an interview with the *Courier-Express*. "We want to see them get better sanitary conditions," Mark declared. "But no one has ever come to us." This was a lie, as the *Courier-Express* detected, writing that Mark "revealed" his earlier correspondence with Dickson later in the interview. The district president continued, "They've gone so far with outsiders I don't know what we could do about the mess now."[17] He made similar remarks to the *New York Post*.

Elizabeth Gurley Flynn of the *Daily Worker* was unpersuaded. She wrote, "If the miners wait for Lewis . . . they'll wait another forty years. He's got a bath, toilet, and running water in Alexandria, Va."[18]

The other telegram recipient, Governor Martin, got off easier. Content to leave matters with his deputy health secretary, the governor seems to have made no reply. That may have disappointed Sprigle, who considered Martin a close friend. A committed Republican and one-time appointee to a patronage job in Allegheny County, Sprigle didn't hesitate to criticize members of his own party. In this case, though, he saved his barbs for other targets.

Even as the governor stayed silent, there was big news from another corner of the state government. The Unemployment Compensation Bureau ruled that the miners' work stoppage stemmed from an industrial dispute and, therefore, they could file for benefits. The compensation, twenty dollars a week, would cover only the work-loss period beginning August 20. The checks would stop after twenty weeks even if the strike was still in effect. At least for a time, mining families would know they could eat.

This small triumph was immediately quashed. Before even one check was cut, Shawmut sent a telegram to the bureau, protesting the ruling and announcing its intent to appeal. Sharing the wired message exclusively with the *Courier-Express*, which presented it without comment, the company demonstrated its distrust in big-city journalism. The DuBois paper had settled into a Twitter-like function in the big local story, content to print accusations hurled by one side without seeking a response from the other.

The telegram, addressed to the bureau director, denied that the company was obligated to provide a doctor. It had been the "practice over many years" to do so by taking "authorized" payments from the miners' paychecks, Shawmut acknowledged, but there was "no agreement." The company had given union officials the names of eighteen "reputable and competent" physicians—only to follow past practice, the message said—but no action had been taken.

The telegram sought to weaponize Hayes's sense of moral responsibility. Shawmut denied that the miners had no physician on hand because "although Doctor Hayes has threatened to leave the community, she has continued to serve the employees and others in the community." Enclosing the telegram in a letter to the *Courier-Express*, Shawmut added one last statement, which the paper printed: "Dr. Hayes continues to occupy the medical quarters provided by the company and holds office hours there." It was the first hint of plans for eviction.[19]

There'd be no checks, at least until a hearing could be scheduled. As the calendar changed to September, the situation seemed to have reached a stalemate. Despite its vague promises of support, the UMWA had done nothing. Pentz, still believing the contract could be reopened, announced his intention to contact union officials. In the meantime, the *Post-Gazette* reported that the miners' committee planned to meet with their Brandy

Camp counterparts, who were still working at Shawmut's Elbon No. 5 mine.[20] However, if this meeting ever occurred, there were no reports of the outcome. News outlets, including Sprigle's paper, continued to name Force, Byrnedale, and Hollywood as the only striking towns, and estimates of the number of idle miners held steady at three hundred and fifty.

Either responding to Pentz or following Lewis's instructions, James Mark met with the miners' committee on September 4. The meeting, reported in the press, produced no official announcement. In the strike's first week, Mark had supported the miners' insistence to let Hayes or "any other interested persons" take part in negotiations. With the men now in their eighth week of a strike about noncontractual issues, Mark may have asked them to reconsider.

Whatever happened at the meeting clearly left Hayes's staunchest allies uneasy. Within days, they were collaborating on another telegram addressed to a powerful recipient. For this project, they retreated to the Hayes family's hunting camp in Medix Run, ten miles from Force. Even there, they couldn't escape the prying eyes of F. J. Erich. The company cop, an avid hunter, evidently followed them into the woods to watch their comings and goings.

Ray Sprigle was present. Not just filing stories, he was "holding forth" at the doctor's camp, according to company intelligence reports. Those reports, of tremendous interest to receiver Dickson, were likely accurate. The telegram conceived at the hunting lodge bore all the hallmarks of Sprigle's distinctive style. Many phrases—about "sewage-sodden" "plague spots" overseen by a "dubious," "suspicious," and "feudal" receivership—were lifted verbatim from his reporting.

His three-part "Plague Spots" delivered a jolt, which had since been absorbed. Despite Sprigle's care to name all the parties, including the three federal judges responsible for overseeing Shawmut's finances in bankruptcy court, no one had been held accountable. The new telegram aimed to change that. Addressed to U.S. Attorney General Tom C. Clark and copied to President Truman, it began,

> We, American citizens residing in the feudal coal company towns of Force, Byrnedale, and Hollywood, appeal to you for justice. We ask that you institute an investigation of the receivership that for 40 long years has administered the bankrupt Pittsburgh Shawmut and Northern Railroad and its subsidiary, the Shawmut Mining Company.[21]

It went on to charge the receivership with its failure to file the financial documents ostensibly demanded by the court. The sanitation woes of

Force, Byrnedale, and Hollywood were quickly summarized with a brief reference to Hayes and her statement about mixing baby formula with urine and fecal matter. The message concluded,

> The three judges of the United States District Court in Pittsburgh have been on notice of these conditions for nearly two months and have taken no action to terminate or even investigate this dubious receivership. We realize that the Federal Government has no authority to abate reeking privies, no matter how noisome, but it does have the authority to investigate courts and suspicious circumstances attending United States receiverships. We the men, women, and children of the sewage-sodden towns of the Shawmut Mining Co., appeal to you for action which will smash this reign of oppression and neglect and restore the American way of life to our people.[22]

Sprigle was not one for subtlety. But if those last lines sound hyperbolic now, they probably didn't then. After four years of fighting against fascism, the nation was ripe for appeals that evoked its founding principles. As Shawmut manager Frank Lambert noted, Hayes had organized the miners like the thirteen colonies.

As with those colonies, there had always been internal tensions. It's possible that Hollywood took no part in the meetings at the hunting camp. The president of its local likely didn't even know about this new telegram. Unlike the messages wired to Governor Martin and John L. Lewis, it wasn't presented at a community meeting for approval. Nor did anyone from Hollywood sign it. Despite the "we the people" style of its first and last sentences, the only signatories were four miners: William Agosti, Joseph Shadick, Anthony Coccimiglio, and Norman Winkler. All were from Force.

"Striking miners in the ramshackle company towns of Force, Byrnedale, and Hollywood played out their last card today," began the *Press* report that included the entire text of the telegram. Ignoring what Sprigle had uncovered for a rival paper, the piece continued, "The company contends—and facts bear out the contention—that it is in no financial condition to make any large-scale improvements in the three towns." It added, not entirely accurately, "Even the United Mine Workers admits that."[23]

Actually, no union official had made a statement about Shawmut's capabilities. The DuBois reporter was parsing from the news digest in the September 1, 1945, edition of the *United Mine Workers Journal*, which stated, "The evidence appears to back up Shawmut's contention that it cannot afford to make any major improvements." In aggregating published reports, the Washington-based union paper seemed unaware of Sprigle's series. Its "evidence" came from Chester Potter's earlier financial analysis in the *Pittsburgh Press*, which also allowed Dickson to lowball his salary. While ostensibly stating the union's position, the *Press* was merely quoting itself.

Inarguably, the *Press* was right on some points. It said the union had been "unable to find a way" to help the strikers' families while the company's appeal of their unemployment benefits had worsened their plight.[24]

As the telegram traveled over the wires to the White House and the U.S. Department of Justice, sanitation inspectors returned to Force. They were checking on the progress of their patch-up job. After capping some wells, pouring cement around others, and adding heaping doses of chlorine, the state was eager to wrap things up.

So was Shawmut, as the dithering James Mark soon discovered. The telegram sent to the White House had Dickson in a tizzy. Imagining life without its current comforts—or even spent behind bars—the absentee executive wrote another long letter to the UMWA's Mark, seeking pity, offering some small concessions, and urging the union to betray its members and their physician.

The company was on the ropes and hoping to settle, Dickson revealed. Sanguine throughout his many years of racking up debt, he now described the "critical situation" caused by the "unauthorized strike." The entire clerical staff of the mining company had been placed on half time, he said. The effects on the PS&N Railroad, which normally shipped mainly Shawmut coal, had also been "disastrous," closing the repair shops in Angelica, New York, and laying off rail workers.[25]

Unless the miners returned to work immediately, Dickson wrote, he'd be forced to apply to the court for permission to abandon the properties. Explaining his reluctance to take that step, he pointed not to his salary but to the "very solemn obligation" to prevent more than one thousand employees from being thrown out of work. As long as the miners stayed out, he added, there'd be no money for a single improvement. He confided to Mark "off the record" that state officials had told him that many Pennsylvania mining towns were far worse, so "why, therefore, we should be singled out as the 'goat' is something which I have not been able to fathom."

But he did have a theory. "I am not of a suspicious nature," he assured Mark, "but I cannot help but feel that there is some influence behind Dr. Hayes which has brought about this unfortunate condition. It seems most peculiar to find a newspaper granting such wide publicity to a situation which does not warrant or merit the effort."

Referring to a "certain specific newspaper correspondent," who'd been meeting with Hayes and the miners at the doctor's hunting camp,

Dickson lamented, "They have even gone so far as to attempt to delve into the private affairs of the writer and officials of the Company." Sprigle's delving seems to have had an effect. Dickson informed Mark that he had neither funds nor "borrowing power" to endure a protracted strike. He could no longer print worthless receiver's certificates for unwitting purchasers.

Behind both the newsman and the doctor, Dickson saw a conspiracy. "There is an underlying issue which neither the United Mine Workers nor the employer can condone or permit," he wrote, hinting at "some outside influence with selfish and ulterior motives." Given the tenor of the postwar times, Mark would have understood this as a reference to communism.

Sometime between July and September, Dickson's image of Hayes had changed from siren to comrade, but he consistently saw her as destructive. His letter contained one accusation that likely was true: "It has come to my attention that on one or two occasions, there has been an attempt on the part of a group of miners to hold a meeting for the purpose of passing upon the question of returning to work only to have it taken over by Dr. Hayes." This was practically an echo of the complaint in his first letter to Mark, when he described how a group of miners had canceled plans to meet with management, apparently after Hayes had put her foot—and her black bag—down. The united front of miners presented to the press had always been fragile. Lately, the cracking had been audible.

On the last page of three single-spaced pages, Dickson made what he obviously considered a generous concession. If the men went back to work, he'd consider negotiating the fines due to the company for the unauthorized strike. He felt sure that if an "honest and uninfluenced" vote were taken, a "great majority" of the men would decide to return to work, and he didn't want the prospect of fines to be a deterrent.

Scattered over the letter were repeated cautions that it was "off the record," "personal," and "to be treated as confidential." It closed by reminding Mark that a meeting between miners and management, *sans* Hayes, could be arranged verbally. Dickson wrote that his mine manager, Lambert, was willing to meet "unofficially" with the miners' committee, adding that Lambert had extended this invitation to Harry Askey, a UMWA District 2 board member.

No reply from Mark has been preserved in the District 2 office files. It's possible that he didn't think the receiver's letter merited a reply. As for the back channel of communication that Lambert was trying to establish, there's no way to know if Askey, a former national organizer for the union, welcomed or ignored it.

For whatever reason, Mark seems to have respected Dickson's wishes for confidentiality. If the contents of the letter had been shared with the miners' committee, the information probably would have reached Sprigle. With a little investigation, he would have found that Dickson was doing far worse damage than cutting workers to half time. Many clerical employees in St. Marys hadn't been paid for weeks. As for layoffs of rail workers in St. Marys, where the Shawmut Line was a major employer, the effects were being felt but not yet reported. The city had a newspaper, the *Daily Press*, but Shawmut's small-town ministry of information had muzzled it. A company that stopped a Pittsburgh paper from crashing the city limits could also censor local coverage. Shawmut had built a wall around St. Marys.

With his talent for forging an emotional connection with readers, Sprigle might have exposed the human cost of Dickson's intransigence. The lives of hundreds of non-miners were being affected by his refusal to deal with Hayes, whom Shawmut now saw as part of a nefarious conspiracy. As the debts owed to shareholders and certificate owners mounted, Dickson was plunging the companies under his care into catastrophe. It would have been a tantalizing story but, then again, journalism had done all it could. The situation called for an investigation, not just investigative reporting.

The deadlock hadn't dampened the public's fascination with Hayes. Katherine Scarborough of the *Baltimore Sun* paid a visit to Force around this time. A longtime feature writer for the paper, she was less interested in filth and finances than in examining the community's connections to the doctor. Much of what she wrote about Hayes's life and local conditions had already been reported, and she made no mention of the White House–destined telegram. Yet Scarborough, who, like Hayes, was professional and single, cast some new light on the subject.

Her feature began, "In the unwritten history of labor relations, women have the reputation of stopping strikes, not starting them." That statement ignores decades of female activism in the needle trades, textile work, and other industries, as well as prominent labor figures like Hayes's champion, Elizabeth Gurley Flynn. But Scarborough meant the wives of strikers. In Force, she wrote, they, like their husbands, were in an "endurance contest with the company."[26] That was true enough.

Probing for fissures, the Baltimore paper couldn't easily find any. A wife with heart disease spoke of Hayes's attentiveness to her during a long illness. A miner credited Hayes with delivering his first child after his wife had suffered six miscarriages. Another showed Scarborough his scarred finger, sewed up by Hayes after he "mashed" it and now nearly good as new. "Without exception, the miners and their families think the world of Dr. Betty," Scarborough wrote, crediting this to the doctor's roots in the community, her competence, and a "talent for human relationships." Perhaps revealing her own class prejudices, the reporter continued, "For all her education, she has never shown the smallest sign of being 'high hat.'"

Scarborough also spoke to Hayes's mother. Anna Hivick Hayes, now living in her new Brockway house, was seldom quoted in the press, maybe because no one interviewed her. She told the *Sun* reporter, "My daughter is a born crusader. Once she gets an idea she thinks is right in her head, she never gives up."

For the sake of balance, Lambert was interviewed. As always, he depicted the strike as a blinking contest, replaying his old standard: "We'll have to see who gets tired of waiting first," to which Hayes replied, "We can hold out as long as the company can."

The *Sun* feature was an admiring profile of Hayes, no different from many others except for one accidental revelation. After chatting with miners and their families, Scarborough produced this startling sentence: "'We ought to be digging coal. The country needs it,' says a spokesman for those opposing the walkout, but still strong for Dr. Betty." Like many other sources for this *Sun* feature, the speaker is unnamed.

If those "opposing the walkout" were organized enough to have a spokesman, the waiting game could soon be over.

6

THE FEDS AND THE GOON

Sending a telegram to President Harry S. Truman was like floating a message in a bottle. The president received three truckloads of mail a day.

Yet within hours of its receipt at the White House, the operatic plea from Force found an audience. Abridging its excesses into a six-line précis, a presidential secretary forwarded it with the note, "Respectfully referred to the Department of Justice."[1] The *Pittsburgh Post-Gazette* was first to report this greased-lightning response, adding that the probe would be handled by the DOJ's criminal division. The scoop ran under its Washington correspondent's byline, not Sprigle's.[2]

Without Ray Sprigle, however, there might never have been a story. The presidential secretary who plucked the message from the mailroom ocean and steered it toward the DOJ was William D. Hassett. "Tall, scholarly" Bill Hassett, as he was described by one journalist, was himself a former newsman. He'd served in the Roosevelt administration as an assistant to Stephen T. Early, filling in at press conferences when necessary.

Hassett may not have met Ray Sprigle, but he would have remembered Sprigle's award-winning series on U.S. Supreme Court Justice Hugo Black. Black's first year on the court had caused multiple headaches for Roosevelt's staff. The president nominated Black, then a U.S. senator from Alabama, without informing his press secretary. While Steve Early was telling reporters about a long list of potential candidates, a messenger was submitting Black's nomination to the Senate. Hassett's boss emerged with egg on his face, which for a while became a story in itself.

Then, a few weeks after Black's 1937 confirmation, Sprigle's series about the new justice's Klan membership during the 1920s set off a political earthquake. Several senators expressed regret for voting to confirm Black, and there were calls for his resignation or impeachment. Protests erupted in front of the new justice's home, rattling him badly. But the tremors eventually subsided, and Black was now a widely respected member of the Court's liberal wing.

A devoted FDR loyalist, Hassett couldn't have been pleased by Sprigle's exposé, but he may have respected or even admired it. It's possible that he blamed Black more than the journalist for the public relations nightmare triggered by the *Post-Gazette*. Leaving Black to defend himself, Roosevelt departed for the West during the height of the controversy. One of Black's biographers wrote, "FDR suggested, through his aides, that he'd been deceived by the Alabaman."[3] One of those aides was Hassett, who eventually left his press duties to become Roosevelt's correspondence secretary.

He did the same in the Truman administration, sorting through the avalanche of letters and telegrams, then reading and responding to them. The miners' message rose quickly to the top, maybe because Hassett was looking for it. Once the telegram was forwarded, the attorney general snapped into action. The feds were coming to Force.

In DuBois, the *Courier-Express* had time to reprint the scoop on its front page, crediting a "Washington correspondent" without naming the *Post-Gazette*. For a half-century, the DuBois daily had been a morning paper, but now it appeared in the afternoon. The newspaper workers had rebelled against the late hours required for an early edition. Like many other workers, they were in a strong bargaining position; the labor shortage had persisted beyond the war.

The need for physicians was still acute. More than 15,000 doctors were awaiting their release from military service. Shawmut, however, had not given up on replacing Hayes. While the federal probe into Dickson's receivership began, Shawmut ran its final ad for a company doctor in the *Journal of the American Medical Association*. As Hayes and the miners sat on the applications already submitted, the company proceeded with its own plans.

The wheels of justice resumed their slow pace. A pair of strangers installed themselves inside the Rogan Building in St. Marys, where various divisions of the PS&N Railroad and its mining subsidiary occupied two floors. But if that town's newspaper, the *Daily Press*, heard about these interesting visitors, it printed nothing about them.

With nothing new to report in early September, the wire services and other Pittsburgh papers turned their attention elsewhere. The only news from Force was another visit from U.S. Representative Leon Gavin, who suggested that the state legislature pass special laws if necessary to correct the situation. Again calling conditions "deplorable," Gavin seemed to wash his hands of them. Even as the executive branch of the federal government launched an investigation, he reiterated his position: sanitation was a state matter that the U.S. Congress was helpless to address.

This time, Gavin's calls for action were aimed at the legislature, not Governor Martin. Hugely popular in the state Republican Party, Edward Martin would eventually be drafted to run, successfully, for the U.S. Senate. Although lacking a crystal ball, Gavin may have sensed political danger in crossing the governor, whose health department had declared its work finished. However, the congressman's return to the coal patch seemed sincere in its intentions. Likely prompted by the invitation of Hayes and the mining families, it at least reflected his interest in his constituents. Gavin represented Force and Byrnedale, but not Hollywood.

Following Gavin's visit, a reporter sought comment from Hollywood's congressman, but was unable to locate him. U.S. Representative D. Emmert Brumbaugh was the winner of a special election. He was saving the seat for his predecessor, a fellow Republican who left Congress for the navy but returned to run for another term. Destined to become a state banking secretary, Brumbaugh had little incentive to visit a remote corner of his district. Hollywood was out of the loop again.

Around this time, Woody Guthrie finished his song about Betty Hayes, giving it the alternate title of "The Company Town Doctor," as well as "The Dying Doctor." The secondary title could have reflected the story's progression as Betty stepped out of Leo's shadow. As is evident in the lyrics, Guthrie had followed the story at least to the point where a state inspector visits Force and declines an offered glass of water. The song ends with the company suffering a self-inflicted loss of thirty thousand tons of coal.

By now, those losses totaled fifty thousand tons, but Guthrie had a lot of other news to follow. He added the descriptor "Documentary No. 1" to his latest album, *Struggle*, because its songs were based on true events. An ad for the album ran in the same issue of the *Daily Worker* that featured the column by Elizabeth Gurley Flynn advising the Force miners not to expect a response from John L. Lewis. Flynn wrote then that no one would have heard of "lonely Bennett's Valley" if it hadn't been for the "gallant stand" of "pretty, blonde Dr. Betty Hayes, who was fortunately good copy for the press."[4]

A new Federal Bureau of Investigation case also made good copy. Press interest revived in mid-September, as Sprigle reported that he had "word from Washington" that federal field agents were looking into the "ancient, hidden and secret ledgers" of the Shawmut receivership.[5] The wire services and other big-city papers held back on this news, unable to confirm it. Then the *Philadelphia Record* learned that Judge Guy K. Bard of the U.S. District Court for the Eastern District of Pennsylvania would be sent to Pittsburgh to hear the case.

As a visitor on the bench at the federal court for the Western District, Bard might well ask why that court failed to demand regular financial reports from the Shawmut receivership. It would be difficult to do so, however, without implying criticism of Judge Frederic P. Schoonmaker of the federal court in Pittsburgh, to whom Dickson was accountable. In what a cynic might call a remarkable stroke of luck, Schoonmaker died in his sleep hours after the Force miners sent off their White House telegram.

Bard, who'd been Pennsylvania attorney general for a brief time, was well known in Philadelphia. His assignment to the Shawmut case inspired another *Record* editorial. This one mentioned Hayes only briefly, focusing instead on the receivership. The *Record* evidently had vetted Dickson through its Manhattan contacts. Sprigle routinely referred to the receiver as a "small-town lawyer," but the Philadelphia paper found no trace of hayseeds. It reported that "John D. Dickson of Wellsville, N.Y., with offices in New York City is known as a very able lawyer." Still, the left-leaning Philadelphia paper found it "odd" that Dickson and McBride over the years, had earned more than half a million dollars for their services while Force and two neighboring towns were denied basic sanitation. Taking a wait-and-see attitude—a marked contrast with its earlier paean to Hayes—the editorial ended, "The whole matter is now to be aired. And none too soon."[6]

The airing metaphor was apt. At the mass meeting, Hayes had advised noncompliance with Shawmut's position that tenants must clean out any toilets that were running over. Since then, a month had passed, and virtually all toilets were in that condition. Still, Hayes said, "It would be better to leave them as they are than to attempt to clean them without proper equipment." She added, "There are state laws which say how such things are to be handled—including the use of covered vehicles, and none are to be found here."[7]

The company suggested the use of hand buckets. As part of what Sprigle called Shawmut's "half-hearted cleanup" to make the minimal changes required by the state, a private contractor had started to clean privies and haul sewage in Hollywood. In Force and Byrnedale, however, rain still produced "trickling rills of sewage," as the miners' ally wrote.[8] The favored treatment of Hollywood echoed the earlier draft-board incident, in which all the inductees happened to come from Force and Byrnedale. At the time, not even Sprigle suspected the danger in that.

After all, there was something to celebrate, even as the strike finished its tenth week with no unemployment checks in sight. Finally convinced by a court filing that a federal probe was underway, the *Pittsburgh Press*—previously more sympathetic than Sprigle's paper to Shawmut's cries of poverty—put the company under its lens again. It reported that two FBI "agent-accountants" had already spent ten days in St. Marys examining "age-yellowed" ledgers to learn how the receivership could "tick along" for four decades while falling deeper in debt.[9]

Meanwhile, a marquee name attached itself to the suit filed by holders of Shawmut's worthless receiver's certificates. Charles J. Margiotti would be an associate counsel for the plaintiffs. Like Judge Bard, Margiotti was a former Pennsylvania attorney general. The addition heightened statewide interest in the case. Bard was scheduled to hear it in Pittsburgh on October 15, when a report from the FBI was also expected.

Pittsburgh would also get another visitor, at least eventually. When the certificate holders sued in 1942, they demanded that Dickson show cause as to why no accounting was made. They also wanted him to explain why the companies under his care shouldn't be reorganized or sold. The federal suit was left pending on condition that it be heard when the war was over. Still ensconced in New York, the receiver would have to find his way to the state line.

For now, Dickson made himself unavailable to the *Press* while other company officials, presumably Lambert and McBride, declined to comment. They could not have been pleased that Pittsburgh's leading newspaper had essentially changed tack, crediting the miners for spurring federal action by sending a telegram to the U.S. attorney general when "all other avenues of relief seemed closed to them."[10] No longer stating that Shawmut couldn't afford town improvements—as if that were an irrefutable fact—the *Press* now presented that as Dickson's position.

The receiver and his underlings had lost control of the narrative in their own bailiwick. For weeks, copies of the *Pittsburgh Post-Gazette* had vanished from St. Marys while the once-friendly *Pittsburgh Press* circulated unimpeded. On a leafy residential street in that city, a grocer named Randolph Soranson took a particular interest in those latest articles in the *Press*. Between waiting on customers and stocking shelves, he clipped the articles from the papers, noting the date in the top margin before slipping them into envelopes for mailing. This was the same man who'd borrowed contraband copies of the *Post-Gazette* to peck out Sprigle's three-part series on a busted typewriter.

For Soranson, it was a labor of love, though it was the Shawmut Line that captivated him, not the mining concern. He'd bought the grocery store, which he operated with his wife, after retirement from his railroad career. A railfan since his youth in Westfield, about thirty miles northeast of St. Marys, he'd spent most of his seventy-two years working for various lines, sending telegrams, auditing reports, and tracking repairs. If a station flooded, he'd grab a mop. The hours were long and the wages low, but his heart was in it.

A talented artist whose illustrations of "odd types of railroad men" were published in a national rail magazine, Soranson for a while worked in Galeton, Pennsylvania, where he owned and edited a weekly newspaper, the *Dispatch*, while performing secretarial duties for the president of the Buffalo & Susquehanna Railroad, F. H. Goodyear. Far from discouraging his assistant's sideline, Goodyear wrote the magazine article that Soranson had illustrated with drawings of "The Pedantic Official" and "The Young Ticket Clerk."

An even better opportunity presented itself when the Pittsburg, Shawmut & Northern line was formed from seven coal roads. Informed by a friend about a secretarial job in the executive office, Soranson abandoned Galeton for the PS&N. The secretarial job quickly disappeared as the new railroad fell into a receivership overseen by New York attorney Frank Sullivan Smith, a close friend of Dickson's father. Reassigned to the freight claims department, Soranson found an outlet for his creativity in designing timetable covers.

Soranson stayed with the PS&N for only a few years. He was there when its mining subsidiary hastily threw up miners' housing in Force and as receiver Smith successfully defended himself against charges of fraud and mismanagement. After working at several other small lines in Pennsylvania and New York State, sometimes helping them close accounts as they went out of business, Soranson left the industry. Sensing where things were going, he sold automotive batteries before buying the market on Center Street in St. Marys.

But his heart was still in railroading, so when approached by a train buff who was preparing a history of the Shawmut Line, Soranson eagerly agreed to help. His news clippings and samizdat transcriptions were destined for Charles F. H. Allen of Rochester, New York. A research scientist for Kodak with a doctorate in chemistry from Harvard, Allen devoted years of his life to the project, eventually publishing several articles about the PS&N and its predecessor lines in the journal of a railway historical society.

It's not clear if the two railfans had ever met. Interviewing other employees for his project, Allen may have obtained the grocer's name and address. Wasting no time on pleasantries, Soranson's letters to the scientist dived right into their shared passion, railroading. Addressing his correspondent as "Mr. Allen" and often signing with only his surname, Soranson supplemented the clippings with typed letters or comments penciled on small notepaper with the Worcester Salt logo.

Allen knew he'd struck gold in discovering Soranson, a train enthusiast with firsthand knowledge of the Shawmut Line's beginnings plus a journalism background. When the two began exchanging letters in 1944, Allen couldn't have known how much he would grow to depend on his pen pal's news instincts. Expecting an old-timer's recollections of the railroad's early days, Allen instead got a front-row seat on current events. With FBI agents examining its books, the PS&N and its mining subsidiary were entering a new phase. Reading any papers he could get his hands on and pursuing local gossip, Soranson kept the amateur historian updated.[11]

He soon had plenty to report. Some of the miners in Hollywood, fed up with the strike, were working with management to reopen the Proctor No. 2 mine. As told to Soranson, "a goodly number" began the last full week of September by cleaning the mine, a necessary step before the resumption of digging. Without consulting their counterparts in Force and Byrnedale, members of the Hollywood local were set to take a strike vote that Tuesday evening. Anticipating a general return to work, the company was readying a train for a run to the coalfields.

But even with lousy phone service, news traveled fast through Bennett's Valley. Committeemen from Force and Byrnedale descended on Hollywood, rounding up men in favor of continuing the strike to make sure they attended the meeting. They also brought Hayes with them. The Force contingent could only stand by as bitter arguments broke out among the Hollywood men in the first part of the meeting. During a recess, Hayes asked to speak, and the men stayed to listen. Sprigle must have been there, too, because he reported all the dialogue word for word.[12]

If the Hollywood miners voted to go back to work, they'd weaken the strike, even if not technically becoming strikebreakers. Although represented on the miners' committee, which traditionally negotiated with management, they had their own UMWA local. As Hayes knew, the effects on the upcoming federal hearing could be disastrous. Judge Bard was looking into the conduct of the receivership, not just its financial mismanagement. If the Proctor No. 2 diggers went whistling back to work, how could the others press their claims of intolerable conditions?

Hayes faced an audience primed for a back-to-work "stampede," as Sprigle called it in his article. Only about forty men had participated in the two-day cleanup, but the company had cleverly arranged it to happen before the Tuesday vote. With its mine prepared, its equipment oiled, and a train scheduled for its siding, Hollywood was ready to roll up its sleeves on Wednesday morning.

Hayes could have begun by chiding the Hollywood men for betraying her. At the start of the strike, she'd declared her intention to leave if the miners tried to settle without her. She chose a different tack altogether. Without shaming anyone, she warned her listeners they could be making a huge mistake by making a deal with the wrong parties. According to Sprigle, the "girl doctor," as he called her, made this prediction: "You can take it as almost a certainty that Dickson and Peter McBride won't even be on the job after the FBI gets through with them. Then you'll have to start all over again with a new management."

A question arose from the seats: "How do you know McBride will be through after the October hearing?" to which Hayes responded, "I don't know. But right here and now, I'll bet you a hundred dollars that both Dickson and McBride will be out." At this point, she "flashed bills," according to Soranson, who summarized this bit of theater in a letter. There were no takers.

It was logical to assume that Hayes had her own sources of information. Hadn't she shined a national spotlight on their valley, even grabbing the attention of the White House? Moreover, she wasn't asking for the moon, just a postponement until the federal court date.

"You've put ten weeks of your time, ten weeks' pay into this fight," she said. "Why not put in 20 days' more pay and time and see what happens?" With that, she left, and the miners took a vote. The outcome was unanimous.

Early the next morning, four men took up their tools and lunch pails and walked to the tipple, where coal would be tipped and loaded into coal cars, already waiting at the siding. This was to be the gathering place for work assignments. They waited for a while, then went home when no one else showed up. As Soranson phrased it in a letter to Allen, the Hollywood miners "finally succumbed and tied up the mine there again."[13]

But one point could have been overlooked in these contemporaneous accounts of the Hollywood meeting. In a magazine interview conducted six months later, Hayes linked this late-September event to the company's announcement that it had found a new doctor. Taking its information from Hayes, the magazine wrote of the aborted back-to-work movement, "At the end of the second day, however, the miners discovered that the new doctor wasn't even licensed to practice in the state of Pennsylvania."[14]

The specificity of the reporting—Hayes had, in fact, addressed the Hollywood local on the end of the second day—suggests that it was accurate. Shawmut had recently stopped advertising for a doctor, accusing Hayes and her allies of failing to consider suitable candidates. In theory, the strikers were not insisting on Hayes's reinstatement to her former job, nor was she necessarily seeking it. In reality, she and her allies knew her leadership was needed to see matters through to a satisfactory conclusion.

If Hayes were replaced, the miners' case for jobless benefits would fold. And without "Dr. Betty," the hearing scheduled for Pittsburgh wouldn't attract much notice. Regardless of licensing or qualifications, no doctor in the world could replace her.

The first half of October was uneventful. Speaking to reporters, attorney Ross Pentz said that Shawmut had shown some rare initiative in its lackluster cleanup effort. While capping some wells and lacing others with chemicals, the company removed the boil-water notices, headed in large capital letters by the warning, "Dangerous!" The state health department had ordered the return of the signs.

Otherwise, the situation was "about the same," the lawyer said, adding, "Everyone seems to be waiting for the outcome of two hearings this month."[15] The federal hearing and the appeal of the unemployment bureau's ruling were scheduled for the same week.

They did not end quite as predicted. No one from Force was invited to the receivership hearing in Pittsburgh, although Judge Bard referred to their plight during the proceedings. The participants were the judge, an attorney for holders of receivers' certificates, and John D. Dickson, making a rare appearance south of the state line.

As it turned out, the Hollywood miners should have taken Hayes up on her bet. Dickson was still the receiver when he returned to Wellsville, New York City, or Buffalo, where he also claimed to be wrapped up in business. But he left with a heavy homework assignment: the judge had ordered him to produce forty years of annual financial statements for the PS&N Railroad, dating from 1905, its first year in receivership.

All clerks remaining in the railroad's workforce, unpaid and hollowed out, would finally have plenty to do. The judge gave Dickson three weeks to produce the reports.

The next steps seemed uncertain. The lawyer for the certificate holders had asked for Dickson's removal. Although that hadn't happened, it was still possible. But Hayes's predictions about the fortunes of McBride and Dickson "when the FBI got through with them" got a splash of cold water. The FBI report showed that the books were "kept in a proper manner as far as it can be ascertained," said the judge, while adding, "I do think it constituted negligence not to have reports filed with the court in all these years."[16]

Clearly, this was not the stuff of gangster movies. Nevertheless, President Truman and his attorney general were interested in this case, as was evident even in this dry hearing. Dickson protested that the coal production of his company had dropped between 1941 and 1944. Judge Bard had a meaningful reply: "No business can be operated profitably without the good will of the employees, and certainly nobody would want to operate any business at the expense of unhealthy sanitary conditions."[17] On that hopeful note, the hearing was adjourned to November 27.

The Hollywood miners had sacrificed twenty more days of work without seeing the promised change of management. For the time being, though, there was no more talk of reopening mines. All attention was focused on the next hearing, the one about unemployment compensation. It would take place closer to home, in Ridgway, the Elk County seat. An attractive community with gracious homes and Italianate commercial buildings, Ridgway held the county courthouse where McBride had been an associate judge. His duties as assistant receiver for Shawmut apparently weren't too taxing, as he'd held both jobs simultaneously.

As extensive as McBride's tentacles were, they didn't quite reach into the hearing that Friday before the state Unemployment Compensation Bureau's Board of Review. The referee in charge of the case was Harvey J. Berkhouse, an attorney from Kane, outside of Elk County. Appointed by former Pennsylvania governor Arthur James, who'd been his law school classmate, Berkhouse had six years' experience hearing cases in north-central Pennsylvania.

McBride wasn't even present. Lambert represented the company, while William Agosti spoke for the miners and Ross Pentz appeared as their counsel. Hayes was there as well. It might have been the first time she had laid eyes on James Mark unless she'd crossed paths with him in DuBois. The president of the UMWA's District 2 was making a rare appearance in connection with the strike at Force.

Testifying before the referee, Lambert refrained from the cocky and extravagant statements that the press had come to expect from him. There were no silly arguments denying that the miners had no medical care because Hayes had continued to practice privately. Appealing the bureau's decision that the men were jobless due to an industrial dispute, Lambert maintained that they'd quit voluntarily. At the heart of his argument was the union contract's silence on housing and medical care.

Lambert also added a new wrinkle. On the first day of the strike, July 16, he said a group of miners had agreed to discuss possible "adjustments" in a meeting with management. But because the miners insisted on having the doctor present, the meeting never happened. Hence, he argued, the men were wrong to walk out. They hadn't exhausted all avenues toward settlement.

Lambert's testimony was the first public disclosure of the aborted meeting. Until now, it was known only to the parties involved and to James Mark, the recipient of Dickson's letter about it. Mark was the next to testify. He confirmed that the contract had no provisions about living conditions. The questions about whether the strike was authorized must have made him uncomfortable. By claiming he knew nothing about the walkout until the Shawmut miners invited him to meet with them, Mark uttered a bald-faced lie. His first letter from Dickson, dated July 25, referred to a letter received from Mark a week earlier. Within four weeks of the strike's inception, he'd been urging management to negotiate with the doctor present.

Why would Mark give false testimony? Possibly just to be consistent with other statements he'd made. The press was at the hearing, and Mark had previously portrayed himself as a helpless bystander who'd encountered the "mess" made of negotiations in Force too late to do anything about it. Truthfully, he told the referee that he'd met with some of the miners in September and offered to set up a meeting with management. Mark added that he advised the miners to return to work but hadn't ordered them to do so.

It was still unclear if Mark had played a part in the thwarted Hollywood back-to-work scheme. Attempting to renew their correspondence, Dickson appeared to view the union official as a potential accomplice. Then again, Dickson was thoroughly self-deluded. Testifying before the Unemployment Compensation Bureau, Mark struck a neutral pose.

If he'd been at the hearing, Dickson might have called out James Mark's fib about when he learned about the walkout. But he was back in New York, and it likely wouldn't have made much difference.

Pentz pointed to a section of the compensation act that provided jobless benefits when workplace conditions were not acceptable to the employees. His filings made mention of the intolerable living conditions, but his presentation stressed the miners' need for a doctor in case of accident or injury.

Testifying about the scotched July 16 meeting with management, William Agosti explained that Hayes had said she "would take her bag and leave" if the men returned to work. This was the first public indication of any tensions between the miners and their physician, whom the press saw as indivisible. Indeed, *Pittsburgh Press* headlines habitually referred to the men as the "'Dr. Betty's strikers." Now it was revealed that Hayes had used strong medicine to include herself in a situation beyond the bounds of collective bargaining.

The AP report on the hearing included Agosti's comment, but didn't play it up. Had it been known in the early days of the strike, the doctor's threat might have seemed startling. But no one was paying attention then, and now Hayes was a celebrity, still getting fan mail by the bagful. It was unimaginable to think of the miners proceeding without her.

Hayes confirmed Agosti's version of events, doubtlessly knowing what he'd say. His testimony was the key point in the miners' unemployment case. With that, the hearing concluded. Berkhouse promised he'd rule as soon as possible.

As the strike entered its fifteenth week, the waiting must have been agony, although less for some than others. Fewer than two-thirds of the strikers—221 miners—were awaiting unemployment checks. Many had found other work, intending to return to mining when the strike concluded. Still, the outcome would affect them all. Without benefits, it would be hard to sustain the strike at this critical juncture when the receivership was under fire.

Ray Sprigle was away during this lull. He was spending several weeks at a New Mexico ranch, preparing to ride along with cowboys on a three-hundred-mile cattle drive over mesas and canyons. Not pegged to any news event, the assignment was apparently a gift to a valued reporter. It would also help fill the *Post-Gazette's* "daily magazine," a section of features, celebrity gossip, puzzles, and comics—the best it could do without a Sunday edition. After months in the fetid air of Force, Sprigle and his Stetson hat were under the open skies of the American Southwest.

Even as nothing in particular happened, Hayes suffered no lack of attention. Somewhat belatedly, two national women's publications took note of her struggle. Along with its usual notes about job promotions, government appointments, and marriages, the *Medical Woman's Journal* reprinted part of the profile written by Elaine Kahn for the Associated Press. Around the same time, the national magazine of Hayes's college sorority, Alpha Omicron Pi, devoted a full page to a reprint of the *Philadelphia Record* editorial with three of the *Record*'s photos of Force. In an introduction to the editorial, the magazine wrote, "Dr. Betty gives a challenge to all AOΠs: "Rx: Get good and mad—and start fighting."[18] These publications offered a chance for women to inspire each other. Hayes, who'd joined groups for professional and university women, must have appreciated the support.

There was also praise, unsolicited and perhaps unwanted, from a more controversial source. Urging all "progressive people everywhere" to support the Force miners in their right to draw unemployment, the *Daily Worker*'s Sunday magazine ran another lengthy article about their "pioneering" struggle against inhuman conditions. For once, Hayes wasn't mentioned by name. The thrust of the piece was the hardship suffered by the miners in enduring a three-month strike without the support of the UMWA.[19]

The Communist Party USA had seized on the benefits hearing as another chance to skewer John L. Lewis. The love letter to the Force miners appeared beside a story accusing Lewis of collaborating with coal operators. According to the piece, the UMWA president was pressing anthracite miners to speed up production. Predictably, the paper harked back to 1943, when Lewis's nationwide strikes had earned Hitler's approval.

Now, there was a different enemy, at least in the minds of some, and association with the *Daily Worker* was growing more perilous. Its managing editor, Louis Budenz, had recently quit his job and rejoined the Catholic Church. He'd publicly renounced communism, declaring that it was irreconcilable with Catholicism. The paper's editorial board rejected this as nonsense, asserting that Budenz's "frightened abandonment of the cause of the labor movement" had nothing to do with religious conviction, sincerity, or courage.

The editorial didn't explain what it meant by "frightened," but an endorsement by the communist paper had recently become more perilous than ever. As pressure on American party members intensified, the Communist Party USA had moved farther from the mainstream, abandoning a short-lived attempt to broaden its appeal. Calls for the party to align itself less closely with the Soviet Union had been rejected. Internal tensions had led to the ouster of the party's former president, Earl Browder, and a new national committee was formed. Among the survivors of the shake-up, or purge, were Roy Hudson and Gabe Kish, coauthors of the latest *Daily Worker* paean to the Force miners.

Hudson had been a Communist Party leader since the 1930s. Kish was elected to the national committee under the name George Kane. The alias would be disclosed years later when a Pittsburgh FBI agent submitted information to the House Un-American Activities Committee about Hudson, Kish, and hundreds of other suspected "reds" in Western Pennsylvania.

When the FBI "got through" with Dickson, in Hayes's words, they found nothing incriminating. The writers of the Communist Party's ode to Force were not so lucky. No miners were quoted or consulted in the communist plea for their jobless benefits, which essentially was an opinion piece. Still, attention from this quarter couldn't have been desirable.

It didn't do any immediate harm, however. Two days after the piece ran, referee Berkhouse upheld the bureau's previous decision: that the miners were entitled to unemployment compensation. Shawmut had failed to convince him that the conditions leading to the walkout didn't constitute an industrial dispute. In the section of the law regarding such disputes, the referee said, "No mention is made of a failure to negotiate a dispute according to the terms of a binding agreement, nor whether or not it covers an outlaw strike." Citing the words "or should any local trouble of any kind arise at any time," Berkhouse continued, "We are of the opinion . . . that this clause is broad enough to cover living conditions and medical service at the mines."[20]

The opinion included a swipe at the winning side: "Publicity given this case in the press paints a sordid picture of the living conditions in the area in controversy, but the testimony discloses only 'intolerable conditions' without further description."[21] When not splitting hairs about the definitions of "sordid" and "tolerable," Harvey Berkhouse was reading the papers.

With that, the miners became eligible for twenty-five dollars weekly per household. Even with the five-week penalty, they could expect ten retroactive pay envelopes. Going forward, they'd be eligible for ten more.

November started on an optimistic note. The mail brought some miners a sheaf of checks. Many accounts were settled at independent stores. Still, there was anxiety; the law stated that "any party" to the case had ten weeks to appeal the ruling again. For now, the company was quiet, but the other shoe could drop. And even if Shawmut couldn't sway Berkhouse, the company didn't entirely lack influence with his bureau. The checks never seemed to arrive at certain houses—the ones occupied by the strike leaders.

Back from New Mexico, Ray Sprigle remained in Pittsburgh, finishing his six stories on cowboys in the New West. The paper promoted the series, promising "a rip-rarin' account of the autumn roundup" with "bucking broncos" and "howling coyotes." However, the stories were mostly a bust. Sprigle's lively style couldn't disguise the fact that a promised three-hundred-cattle drive failed to materialize. Instead, a California buyer put in a huge order, and the cowboys stayed on the ranch to load animals onto trains.

Talented at translating obscure trade jargon into conversational language, Sprigle managed to fill the pages with observations about horse breeding and cattle prodding. He'd used the same gift to guide readers through Shawmut's decades of financial entanglements. But there were no injustices to expose at New Mexico's Bell Ranch, and if the cowhands "risk[ed] their lives a dozen times a day" on the cattle drives, as Sprigle wrote, they didn't do so while he was there, waiting for one to start.[22]

It wasn't his kind of story. According to former colleagues, he preferred ones that involved challenges and risks, especially if it was about something wrong. So when the spotlight swung around to Dickson again, Sprigle interrupted his accounts of campfires and cow ailments to cover developments. There was no need for him to revisit Bennett's Valley; the action had shifted to the federal court in Pittsburgh, where Dickson had submitted forty years of financial reports to Judge Bard.

The temperature was rising. Dickson was ordered to show cause why he should not be removed as receiver. Accounting submitted by the company showed more than $30 million in losses since the start of the receivership. In response, the judge had allowed the filing of a petition by holders of receiver's certificates. First filed three years earlier but delayed because of the war, this petition did more than ask Dickson to show cause. It called for his removal.

A hearing was scheduled for November 27, two days before Thanksgiving. Unlike the earlier session at which Dickson received his homework assignment, this would be an open hearing. For Hayes and the strike leaders, it would be a first face-to-face encounter with their tormenter. It wasn't yet clear who could give testimony. The petitioners were Albert Russ of Reading and Albert Schlager of Lehigh County. Schlager was a business booster and sports enthusiast in the Allentown area. An immigrant from Romania, he had recently built a large bowling complex in the small town of Slatington, on the site of his former dry goods store. Lacking Dickson's blueblood pedigree, Schlager compensated with drive and energy. The coal-and-rail past had met the bowling-alley future.

Among the reasons listed by the petitioners for Dickson's removal was that "his administration caused widespread criticism," an obvious nod to the media interest in conditions in the mining towns. The petition charged the receiver with "reckless disregard of his duty" to preserve the value of assets of properties. Failing to make a reorganization plan, they said, he'd continued to do business while "ignoring heavy operating losses year after year."[23]

A federal agency was about to assess the damage. By order of Judge Bard, the Reconstruction Finance Corporation would have access to all of the receivership's properties and books. In control of government loans to railroads and other businesses, the RFC would decide if Dickson's handiwork was worth salvaging with federal aid.

The judge's orders were widely reported, leading to speculation in St. Marys about the future of the Shawmut Line. Soranson, the St. Marys grocer, mailed news clippings to the railroad's self-appointed historian, with a note describing the local reading of the situation:

> Mr. Allen
>
> Some of the latest understood from talks last night with a prominent employee. This office force and some other employees have received no pay for services for about 2 months or more. General opinion here is that Dickson and others will be relieved of management and there are divergent views as to disposition of property. Some think the P&SRR or PRR will take over, mainly the former.[24]

The "P&SRR," as Soranson wrote it, was the Pittsburg & Shawmut Railroad, which was independent of the Pittsburg, Shawmut & Northern Railroad, despite its similar name and spelling. The two shared common origins but had split apart in 1916. Confusingly enough, both were still nicknamed the Shawmut Line and had similar green logos. Operating to the south of the PS&N, the P&S was also a short line. The "other" Shawmut Line ran trains between Brockway and Freeport, close to Pittsburgh. Conceivably, the former sibling could benefit by extending northward instead of paying other lines to carry its freight.

The other putative suitor, the PRR, was a different story altogether. This was the Pennsylvania Railroad or "Pennsy," one of the nation's major transportation companies with thousands of miles of rail lines. As Soranson indicated in his note, rumors of its interest in Dickson's ailing receivership fell into the category of wishful thinking. The mighty Pennsy, facing challenges from trucking, probably didn't need to buy a headache.

The railroad employee at the source of these rumors was taking a risk by confiding in Soranson. Then again, few in St. Marys were likely to know of his correspondence with a writer in Rochester. Slight of build and elderly, the grocer made an unlikely spy. In St. Marys, though, transmitting local gossip was the practical equivalent of espionage. Pumping customers for information as he served them at the counter—self-service was not yet customary—Soranson collected tidbits and recorded them. It was the only form of newsgathering possible in St. Marys, where Dickson had muzzled not only his employees but also, as was later discovered, the local press.

Stung by the federal court, Shawmut was determined to strike back. Its accomplice, probably an unwitting one, was an applicant for the company physician position. Even as Dickson prepared for the legal fight of his life, he wasn't too busy to plot against Hayes.

The ideal candidate had emerged, complete with a medical degree and Pennsylvania license. Indeed, his application was so unassailable that the miners had to go through the motions of considering it. Dickson wasn't out yet, and the company could still file another appeal to the unemployment bureau.

Definitions of industrial dispute aside, the miners would have a hard time defending the walkout if provided with this physician. Shawmut had one more shot at getting even with Hayes and halting the unemployment checks, which still hadn't reached the four biggest troublemakers: Bill Agosti, Tony Coccimiglio, Joseph Shadick, and Frank Winkler. Even the name of this prospective savior seemed to guarantee a cure: Dr. Charles Tonik.

A naturalized U.S. citizen with Russian Jewish roots, Tonik had attended medical school under the name Charles Tunitsky. Like Hayes's father and uncle, he attended the Medico-Chirurgical College in Philadelphia, graduating in 1915, shortly before its consolidation into the University of Pennsylvania School of Medicine. Two years later, he obtained his Pennsylvania license under his new surname and served an internship at a hospital in Chester.

No stranger to coal communities, Tonik had been the company doctor for a mining concern in Brush Valley, west of Allentown. Subsequently, he'd moved to Philadelphia with his wife and two sons, setting up private practice there. It wasn't clear how he had spent the war years, but he sent his application to Shawmut from Raleigh, North Carolina, where he was living at the time.

At fifty-five, he was past the age when most professionals start a new job in a new location. Then again, he and his wife were no strangers to Pennsylvania. Before his first coal town job, he'd lived in Pittsburgh. He even worked for the state health department for a time, inspecting schools in the area around Mechanicsburg, where he and his wife had their first child. The one possible blot on his resume was his frequent change of residences, although perhaps that could be explained. As for his age, he was still nine years younger than Dr. Leo Z. Hayes had been when suddenly killed by a brain abscess.

Shawmut probably didn't know that Tonik had testified, at least once, in support of an injured employee's claim for workers' compensation benefits. In 1931 the doctor served twice as a witness for a riveter, maintaining that an accident had left the man too disabled to perform his job. Other physicians testified that the disability was negligible and that the man was disguising his improvement. The referee awarded the injured man a small sum for what he judged temporary and partial impairment.

A coal company involved in such a case would want its doctor to testify against the employee. But Tonik's involvement in the case was separate
from his mine employment: the injured man worked for an oil refinery.
Giving testimony as a private physician, Tonik was probably looking for
some extra income. The workers' compensation case, heard in Philadelphia, was just one part of a varied career that had brought him to many
locations.

Hoping to make Force his next stop, Dr. Tonik came to the area
at Shawmut's invitation. It's unclear where he stayed but, as Sprigle had
pointed out, McBride lived in a roomy St. Marys "mansion." If the visiting
physician failed to suspect that he was stepping into a hornet's nest, then
he wasn't a man who read the papers. A stay in St. Marys, a news desert,
wasn't going to enlighten him.

In the company's mind, Tonik was "the new man" already, but
Shawmut went through the formality of notifying Pentz, probably because
the attorney represented the miners' committee. Soliciting the miners' approval on the hiring of a doctor was an established practice, not only in
Bennett's Valley but elsewhere in UMWA District 2.

Knowing that the days of the current management were probably
numbered, Pentz slow-walked the process. Evidently, he relayed some
questions from the miners to Tonik, maintaining the charade of their willingness to accept a replacement for Hayes. He may have also reminded the
company that, by a vote taken at the mass meeting in August, the miners
were not solely in charge of hiring. The responsibility had passed to a citizens' committee that included Hayes.

Wearing his citizens' committee hat, Bill Agosti said he tried to fix a
date and time for Hayes to meet her prospective successor, but she was "so
busy." Hayes, indeed, was almost always seeing patients; however, if Agosti
wanted to find out when she was free, he could just ask one of his siblings.
Since her mother's departure, Hayes had used the big doc's house only as
an office. She slept and ate elsewhere, most likely in the home of Henry
Agosti, a brother of Bill, and his wife, Martha. The couple had a toddler but
no other children. That left them space to accommodate a guest, as well as
time to shop and cook for her. Close friends of Hayes's sister Aileen, Henry
and Martha Agosti were practically family.

Shawmut's private detective, F. J. Erich, would have known of these
living arrangements. It was his job to do so, and even as the company's
workforce in St. Marys shrank from 360 employees to 290, its "pussyfoot"
remained on the payroll. He'd pleased Dickson by disclosing Sprigle's pres-

ence at the strike meetings convened at the Hayes family hunting lodge in Medix Run.

Now he had another chance to prove he was worthy of continued employment. On November 13, Erich drove to Force with an eviction notice for Hayes. The company would have heard that she couldn't be bothered to meet with Dr. Tonik. Humiliated in the press and facing possible financial ruin, Dickson was determined to fight to the last ditch. Shawmut would kick Hayes out of her company-owned office and install the new doctor.

Erich, scouting for Hayes so he could hand-deliver his letter, couldn't have been pleased that it was 10:00 p.m. when he finally encountered her. The excuse she'd given for not meeting with Tonik—her busyness— was based on the truth.

When she took the letter from Erich, Hayes wasn't all that surprised, knowing that the miners had interviewed Tonik. Addressed to her from Frank J. Lambert, the letter said that the mining company wished to take "prompt possession of the premises known as the Doctor's Residence in Force . . . recently vacated by the tenant, Mrs. Leo Hayes."

It's entirely possible that the doctor was confused about the deadline. Traditionally, tenants were given five days to clear out, and the letter was even more specific. It ended by saying, "We respectfully request that you arrange to vacate these offices in this building and on these premises before the close of the week ending November seventeenth."[25] That was a Saturday—for her a day of office hours and house calls.

Regardless of the date, Hayes didn't take the letter seriously. Shawmut had lost its unemployment appeal, and Dickson had been pilloried by a federal judge. Moreover, the letter was framed as a respectful request. Five-day eviction notices were for tenants who were behind on the rent. Hers was all paid up.

She went to sleep at Henry and Martha's house, leaving the big doc's house unlocked, as always.

7

MARAUDERS

Betty Hayes began her Saturday office hours at the big doc's house at 10:00 a.m. and stayed until 1:00 p.m. After that, she followed her usual routine, eating lunch at her lodgings before driving out on house calls. Checking on the progress of a seventy-one-year-old heart attack victim, she diagnosed pneumonia and needed to return to the office for medication. By then it was around 2:30 p.m.

She found a moving van parked outside her door and men loading it with her furniture, medical instruments, and office equipment. Walking inside past Special Agent Erich, who was guarding the door, she recognized two other faces. David Bell, the mine superintendent and her neighbor, was in the house once occupied by Leo Hayes, the doctor who had saved his son's life. Frank Lambert was here from St. Marys.

The two Shawmut officials were ransacking her office, pulling her diploma and license off the wall and handling garments she kept there. As shocked and violated as she must have felt at the time, Hayes was careful with her words. "You realize, of course, that you can't do this according to the law," she told Bell, whom she'd known since she was a child.[1]

Bell smiled and pointed to Erich, hulking in the doorway. "That's the law around here," he said.

Grabbing some medication for her immediate needs, she told Lambert and Bell they would have to leave her access to her medicine and surgical instruments. She informed them that three of the patients under her care were seriously ill, and "out here in the hills, we don't have a drugstore on every corner." The company officials agreed to put them aside.

Acting as if this were a normal moving day, one of the pillagers motioned toward the truck and asked where Hayes wanted her other things taken. The doctor refused to play along. "That's your baby now," she responded.

Finishing her house calls a few hours later, she returned to find the truck gone and her doors festooned with no-trespassing notices. Signed by John D. Dickson, they warned that this land was the private property of Shawmut Mining Company and that any persons found trespassing on it would be fined ten dollars. At least one door, the rear one used by patients, was padlocked.

As Hayes told the papers, it was possible that the medications she wanted to be safeguarded were somewhere inside. Despite the padlock, there was a way to get into the house. But she wasn't going to become a trespasser in order to find out.

According to witnesses, a small crowd had gathered while the raid was in progress. They said a boy had stopped by to pick up penicillin for an older relative, only to be told that he couldn't have it because "the company's putting the doctor out." Others watched their own medical records heaped onto a truck, which someone said was a moving van from St. Marys Transfer Company.

Hearing about the ransacking, Tony Coccimiglio went to the house and confronted Erich, asking for an explanation. Declining to answer questions, Erich said he was just there to see that "no trouble started." Imagining possible scenarios, Coccimiglio changed the subject. Deer hunting season was around the corner, so there was always that.[2]

Erich didn't know how lucky he was. Busy with other things that day, the other members of the miners' committee didn't hear about the raid until later. The one cool head among them was Coccimiglio, who cautioned them to put away their guns. Speaking of the Shawmut officials, he said, "Their own stupidity is doing them more harm than if you used machine guns on them."[3]

Soon afterward, Lambert conveyed a written message to Hayes, stating that the goods and furniture removed from her office were in an engineering building in Byrnedale. Listing the names of three people who had keys, he added, "If you tell us where you wish them delivered, we will deliver them at [sic] the place designated."

Hayes sent a reply: Put them back where you got them. Then she set about the business of hauling Lambert and his cronies into court.

She kept Ross Pentz busy that weekend. Told about the pillaging, he got in touch with Edward J. Blatt, the district attorney for Elk County. Blatt had just been elected to a second four-year term. The party-backed candidate of the Republicans, he'd also won the Democratic primary as a write-in candidate.

"Eddie" Blatt was a well-known figure in Ridgway, where he lived. The son of a Clarion bartender, he was a popular public speaker, often seated on the dais at testimonials. A state official in the Knights of Columbus, he'd served as counsel to that Catholic organization during its drive to ban "indecent" literature. But that was before the war. Now the thirty-eight-year-old DA was engaged in more forward-thinking projects, like a plan to identify and treat mental illness in veterans and civilians.

Speaking to Blatt on the weekend, Hayes's lawyer couldn't have been certain the district attorney would prosecute. As Pentz had told the press, "The company has been running its affairs and the lives of its miners in a feudalistic manner for years."[4]

But Elk County feudalism was fading. Despite McBride's position in the county judiciary, Blatt was willing to go after the two Shawmut executives and their private detective. Whether or not he thought he could win the case, he was willing to try. Indeed, the young prosecutor became one of Hayes's staunchest supporters.

Pentz spent his Sunday drawing up the charges. Lambert, Bell, and Erich were accused of forcibly entering Hayes's office and looting it. An additional clause charged them with "maliciously conspiring together" to accomplish their task. Heading the list of items taken "feloniously" were drugs and instruments. Others were medical books, private papers, a medical diploma, a medical certificate, office equipment, and clothing. In addition to supporting the charge of larceny, the list of items told a story. A doctor responsible for four thousand rural people had been robbed of the tools of her trade.

While Pentz wrote up the charges, Hayes converted the kitchen at Henry and Martha's house into a makeshift examination room. Their parlor, papered with large floral motifs, would be the waiting area.

Early on Monday, she and Pentz went to a justice of the peace in Tyler, another valley mining village, where she was deposed. Charges were filed, and warrants went out for the arrest of Frank Lambert, David Bell, and Francis J. Erich.

The news hit the streets that afternoon in Pittsburgh and DuBois. The spotlight had swung back to Force again. A crime story with a well-known and sympathetic victim, this was made for the front pages. Readers soaking up the sordid details were reminded of the upcoming receivership. Reports on Shawmut's management, laden with figures and dates, had receded to the back pages. The storming of the doctor's office gave them new life.

"It looks now as though a broad streak of insanity has developed in Shawmut's receivership," said Pentz, as reporters and photographers braved the muddy roads of Force, eager to view the padlocked doc's house.[5]

A constable sent to St. Marys served the warrants on Monday. At the advice of Shawmut's lawyer, the three men surrendered themselves that afternoon. Miners who'd hoped to pack a courtroom hearing were disappointed. At 4:00 p.m., they stood before Eugene V. Flynn, the justice of the peace who'd deposed Hayes. Flynn was a dentist in Kersey, a mining village about ten miles from Force. After the deposition, Hayes might have borrowed some of his medicine and equipment. She'd spent much of the day dashing between Brockway and DuBois, scrounging for stethoscopes and pharmaceuticals.

The men were released on a bond of $200 each in Flynn's jurisdiction. Additional bail—$1,000 per man—had to be paid in Ridgway. With that, the case was bound over to a grand jury, to be heard in January. Deprived of blood sport, the miners spent the day in the Force Hotel, where *Pittsburgh Press* reporter Chester Potter joined them at the bar. He'd broken the story about the extraordinary length of the receivership and the magnitude of its debt. It was Potter who had accepted the company's excuses for the shape Force was in.

Not always sold on Hayes's version of events, Potter wrote that a "reporter"—doubtlessly himself—had found an open door in the doc's house with a sign directing her to medicine and instruments on a table inside. Hayes explained that the no-trespass order was equivalent to a lock. Quoting the reply to present her as somewhat unreasonable, Potter seemed to have missed the point. She could have grabbed some swabs and such, but only by breaking into her own office.

Hayes rewarded the *Press* reporter by eluding him during much of his stay in Force. Trying to interview her, he said, was "like trying to skip rope in a revolving door."[6] Unquestionably, she was in near-perpetual motion. Potter described the stream of patients entering her makeshift quarters before she departed to check on a hospital patient and make half a dozen house calls. Mourning the loss of her scalpel, scissors, sutures, and medicines, she said injury cases would probably have to go twenty miles to a hospital. She added that she hoped to be in bed by midnight.

That left the *Press* reporter with the miners at the Force Hotel, where they spent much of the day expressing their outrage. Among them were some young war veterans, frustrated that the company hadn't settled. "We came back home to find we had no jobs," Walter Yonkofski said. "And I fought on Guadalcanal." Another returning service member, Angelo Gagliardi, had read about the strike in the Manila edition of *Stars and Stripes*. "I'd like to have come back to my job," said Gagliardi, who nonetheless was impressed by what Hayes had started. "Jeepers, was I surprised to read about something happening in Force way out there," he said.[7]

Now Shawmut attorney Thomas G. Gregory, pursued by journalists, got his shot at ephemeral fame. Hayes and Pentz separately told reporters that five days hadn't elapsed from the time she'd received the notice to vacate. Hayes added that she hadn't decided how to proceed. Pentz maintained that the minimum notice to vacate business quarters was thirty days anyway. Gregory declared these calculations irrelevant. He said Hayes had indicated that she wouldn't leave anyway.

The company lawyer didn't specify how Hayes had indicated this. If in writing, that evidence was never produced. More likely, it came from Shawmut's usual source of information: its private sleuth, Erich, whose role in the burglary—indeed, in the company—had assumed an aura of mystery. Writing the theft charges, journalists identified the defendants as "two Shawmut officials," Lambert and Bell. They were stumped by Erich, calling him the "third man" or "an employee." Even the attorney for Shawmut was puzzled; in a court filing, Gregory referred to his client as "Defendant Erich [who] was what was known as the Company Detective."[8]

The man who'd described himself as a "special agent" to the U.S. Census was confusing law enforcement officials in Elk County. Long known to mining families as a company-paid detective or police officer, he wasn't officially registered as such. An unbylined piece for the *Post-Gazette*, most likely by Ray Sprigle, commented on Erich's unclear status:

> Since Pennsylvania outlawed the coal and iron police [*sic*] of an earlier day, years ago, Elk county officials agree that Erich can't be a coal company policeman. Best guess of Elk county law enforcement officers is that Erich is a railroad officer for the Pittsburg, Shawmut & Northern Railroad, parent company of Shawmut Coal, but has been performing the duties of a coal and iron policeman of a decade ago.[9]

Sprigle took special pride in articles he'd written sixteen years before about the savage murder of a miner by the Pittsburgh Coal Company's Coal and Iron Police, which in those days were commissioned by the governor. Barcoski's murder inspired a 1935 movie, *Black Fury*, based partly on a short story by a Pennsylvania judge, Michael Musmanno. The well-reviewed film starred the Academy Award–winning actor Paul Muni.

For the many Pennsylvanians familiar with the murder or the movie, the association of Erich with the despised private police forces was hardly flattering. In St. Marys, Randolph Soranson, who was clipping articles about the break-in and arrests for his fellow railfan, grew concerned about Erich. The large man and his wife were frequent customers at his store, and Erich had made a small contribution to railroad history.

When not stalking mining villages, Erich acted as a security guard for the railroad. As such, he'd accompanied Soranson's correspondent, Charles F. H. Allen, to a Shawmut Line curiosity known as the Kasson Loop. Built at tremendous expense, this was said to be the five miles of rail that bankrupted the railroad. Tackling the steep grades between Clermont and Kasson, near Smethport, Kasson was an enormous double loop built into the sides of hills, bringing the front and rear of a train so close that the train seemed to be passing itself.

For Allen, the once-famous "Loop-de-Loop" was an impressive sight, which he described at length in his PS&N history. He immediately remembered the "cop," as Soranson called him, who'd chauffeured him there. Allen asked his pen pal how the case against Erich was proceeding, but Soranson said there'd be no news until January. In the meantime, the grocer's journalistic background couldn't help him pry information from the cop or his wife. He told Allen that both came into the store frequently, but neither wanted to talk about the case.

The Erichs weren't the only ones eager to distance themselves from it. The St. Marys Transfer Company strenuously denied that any of its trucks had carted away property from Dr. Hayes's office. Relying on witness reports, several papers had erroneously associated the vehicle with the moving company, which demanded corrections. The affair smelled to high heaven, and the local business wanted nothing to do with it.

Dr. Tonik took the same attitude. The doctor's house, stripped to make way for his occupancy, stayed vacant. According to Bill Agosti, Tonik suddenly returned to North Carolina, doubtlessly out of concerns for his own health and safety. As the *Pittsburgh Press* summarized the situation, "Miners' Resentment Runs High Over Dr. Betty's Eviction."

"We don't know what to say about him," said Agosti about the vanished doctor. "After all, he's kind of old to be starting out in a strange district." Moreover, the miners weren't impressed by his responses to their questions. "We asked him why he wanted to come out here, and he said to take care of the sick. We want someone who will keep us well but also take care of us when we're sick."[10] His comments were a tribute to Hayes and her relentless focus on wellness.

Agosti was photographed with the piece, along with fellow strike leader Joseph Shadick. Attired in three-piece suits and scrutinizing a document together, the men are identified as members of the "community committee," the newest name for the entity that included Hayes. Neither man looks like he'd ever dug coal or used an outhouse. These individuals were unquestionably capable of choosing their own doctors.[11]

Agosti expressed—or feigned—disappointment at the job hopeful's sudden departure, claiming, "We wanted Dr. Tonik and the company officials to meet with Dr. Betty."[12] The remark was a sly jab at the company. As Dickson had long ago made clear, no Shawmut official would willingly attend a meeting with Hayes present.

Soon the receiver would have no choice. The long-awaited showdown was looming. Judge Bard had invited Hayes and the miners to testify at the receivership hearing. Less than two weeks after her office was invaded, they'd all be together in the same room.

The Thursday before the hearing would be the first postwar Thanksgiving. Americans were free to plan their feasts. Virtually all food rationing had ended except for sugar. But for all sides in the Shawmut case, there was little time to cook or digest.

Preparing for the federal hearing, the miners abandoned all pretense of considering other doctors. They planned to tell Judge Bard that they wouldn't return to work unless Hayes were reinstated. Any testimony they gave in Pittsburgh couldn't just benefit investors. Not satisfied with bit parts in the certificate holders' financial drama, the miners—or rather, the community committee—would present a separate petition.

Their lawyer puckishly called it the Pentz peace plan. Lured back to the Force Hotel by the beer-drinking and card-playing, and the chance for another story, Chester Potter and his photographer took another picture. Posing with a phone held to his ear, the grinning Pentz looked more than professional. He was having a ball. Presumably consisting of three points, the plan was all about Dr. Elizabeth O. Hayes. First, the company had to sit down with her and the miners and work out a method to improve sanitation in the three towns. Second, she'd be reinstated, with the company allowing the union local to take charge of her monthly payments. Finally, if these conditions were met, the men would go back to work.

Having already postponed her departure several times, Hayes had promised the men she would stay until the following summer. In exchange, the men made clear that they'd accept no substitutes. "They won't desert her," said Pentz, preparing to submit his plan to the committee for a vote. "She insists that some real improvements be made in the sanitary conditions so that the health of the men and their families will not be in constant danger. They want that too, and so they are willing to work to get it."[13]

The back-to-work plan mentioned the current receiver by name: "Judge Bard must direct Receiver Dickson to deduct the usual amounts for medical service from the miner's pay and pay the total monthly to the UMW local." Their attorney was preparing for a world that still included Dickson. Even smiling for his press photo, Pentz couldn't be sure about the outcome of the hearing. Nor were they sure how much longer they could hold out. Speaking to the *Press* reporter, Pentz revealed that Hayes was no longer getting any money from the miners for her medical services. "She refuses to take any," he said, and "they want to see that she gets paid."

Unemployment payments varied by case. The miners averaged eighteen dollars weekly. For families without other income, this was welcome but insufficient. Then, too, there was the boredom of living in Force. "The men want to go back to work," said Pentz. "They're not satisfied living off unemployment compensation payments and spending their time hunting. They're interested in getting back on the job."

As he spoke, some men hadn't yet received a cent in jobless benefits. These were four of the union leaders, now self-identified with the community committee: Tony Coccimiglio, Bill Agosti, Joseph Shadick, and Frank Winkler. Their first checks finally arrived on the day before Thanksgiving—too late to be cashed at a bank.

There was another problem. The checks were dated from August, but stamped with the notation that they had to be cashed within sixty days. Far more time than that had elapsed. "A careful bank would hesitate to cash them," said Pentz.

The men immediately suspected Shawmut of pulling some strings with the state Unemployment Compensation Bureau. They had no proof of this, of course, but they had the increasingly sympathetic ear of the *Pittsburgh Press*. They contacted its local stringer, who wrote, "The miners make no secret of their belief that officials of the mining company are using 'political influence' with someone in the state bureau to make it difficult for them to continue the strike."[14]

Never mind that a referee for the bureau had ruled twice in their favor. As Christmas neared, the story about the hard-to-cash checks made Dickson look like Scrooge, just in time for the hearing. It also afforded the *Press* a chance to remind readers that Shawmut was $30 million in the red and that two of its officials had just been charged with burglary.

Dickson had little for which to be thankful that week. As demanded by Judge Bard, he filed court papers arguing against the petition for his removal. These filings were blasted by Albert Schlager, the bowling alley entrepreneur who had sunk money into a certificate of obligation signed by Dickson.

Schlager and his fellow petitioner filed fourteen exceptions to Dickson's report, charging him with "complete destruction of the capital structure of the railroad corporation." Through their attorney, Bernard Goodman, they said Dickson had failed to justify the continuance of the receivership "despite the ever-increasing and continuing losses" and "tremendous depletion and depreciation of assets."[15]

In addition to these allegations of negligence, there was the suggestion of wrongdoing. During all this, Dickson had acquired the capital stock of the Tyler Coal Company. The petitioners wanted to know if he had court approval to do that.

While check-cashing woes were of interest only locally, this news attracted notice in the nation's capital. Inspired by developments in Force, Senator Burton K. Wheeler, chairman of the U.S. Senate's interstate commerce committee, began seeking authorization to investigate all long-term railroad receiverships. "Frankly, I think this receivership business is getting to be a scandal," said Wheeler, a Montana Democrat. "The only reason for them that I can see is that some receivers and lawyers want to draw down fat fees."[16]

For Dickson, still drawing those fat fees, it wasn't a grim week in the least. At a dinner hosted in his Wellsville home, he and his wife announced their daughter Jane's engagement to a veritable Prince Charming. Freshly graduated from Elmira College and working at a Manhattan bank, Jane had accepted the hand of John Arnot Rathbone Jr.

The receiver's prospective son-in-law was an Air Force fighter pilot who'd won nearly every decoration possible. Moreover, as both an Arnot and a Rathbone, he was descended from two of the wealthiest, most powerful families on New York's Southern Tier. In Elmira, the Arnots and the Rathbones had built fortunes in railroads, canals, mills, foundries, and finance. Attacks on Dickson in Pittsburgh had no reverberations in Elmira or the Wellsville Country Club, where the couple planned to host a rehearsal dinner in advance of their January wedding. They would honeymoon in Florida.

In Bennett's Valley, there were fewer options for recreation, as Hayes often said. Teenagers often had nothing to do but hitchhike to the movies.

Or they could walk along the highway. If they went in a group, that seemed safe enough.

On the frigid night that followed Thanksgiving, a bunch of kids from Hollywood went to the Friday night picture show in Penfield. Some of them linked arms on the three-mile walk back home. Joe Marshall, also from Hollywood, was driving in the same direction. He made sure to give them ample room, noticing that a few of these groups had spread into the road.

As he passed one trio, they suddenly swung farther into the road, and he hit them with his right fender. Thirteen-year-old Diana Volpe was dressed for the weather in overalls and a heavy jacket. Part of this bulky outfit caught on Marshall's parking light. Launched into the air, the girl fell heavily on some younger boys, bruising them slightly before her hard landing.[17]

Someone, maybe a flagged-down driver, summoned Hayes from the house where she was staying. She pronounced the girl dead and had her body taken to a funeral home. On Saturday morning, the Clearfield County coroner filled out the death certificate. The cause was a broken neck.

The teenager was said to have died instantly, which may have been of some small comfort to her parents. Said to be a lively girl and a leader among her peers, Diana was her parents' only child. Her father was a coal miner. The funeral was held at St. Joseph's Church in Force, where the family worshiped.

After an investigation, the state police concluded that the driver, a career Navy man, had done everything possible to avoid the crash. It was just a tragic accident. Then again, it might not have happened if Shawmut had accepted Hayes's blueprint for change. She wanted youth recreation in the mining villages, not three miles down an unlit highway.

The next week would determine whether Hayes would ever be heard in these matters. Giving her a voice was the first point in the Pentz peace plan. Essentially, it was the only point.

8

FEET TO THE FIRE

Force was loaded for bear, quite literally, as the next week began. The four-day bear hunting season started on Monday at 7:00 a.m. Hunting licenses were pinned to many a checkered jacket, the preferred outerwear at this time of year for men and women alike.

Instead, Dr. Betty Hayes was packing a fur muff, ruffled blouse, and velvet jacket into an overnight case. At some other houses in town, suits were pulled from hangers. The doctor and three other community committee members—Joe Shadick, Tony Coccimiglio, and Bill Agosti—were expected at the federal courthouse in Pittsburgh at 9:00 a.m. on Tuesday. Because Monday was a full day for Hayes, still seeing patients with borrowed instruments, that meant an overnight trip.

As week 20 of the strike commenced, it was just another day at the Force Hotel bar for many. But now there was a mood of expectancy. The hearing would determine whether John D. Dickson continued as receiver. Even *Business Week* had run a piece about the once-obscure executive and the four-decades-long receivership.[1] The barflies in Force were one step ahead of the national financial pages. They also wanted to be rid of Lambert and Bell, the marauders of the doctor's office.

But the hearing had to change more than the cast of characters. Living conditions had to improve in the three towns. The Pittsburgh court proceedings would decide whether 350 miners and their families had won a struggle that began in July.

The Force Hotel had attracted—or repelled—many news correspondents since. The new face in the barroom was that of Bill Davidson, a former writer for *Yank*, a service magazine. He and other former staffers for *Yank* and *Stars and Stripes* were preparing to launch a new publication for veterans, called *Salute*. Plans for the debut issue included a possible feature about Hayes, whose cause had attracted mail and interest from service members around the globe.

Davidson was here to see how it all turned out. His photographer took shots of Hayes's makeshift office in Henry and Martha Agosti's home. In another photo, a woman lugged a water bucket along a slushy road as two men conversed, their boots submerged in water. There was also a shot of adorable children, described by their father as "brought up on urine."

Not sure if they could paint such pictures in testimony—or even if they'd all be asked to speak—Shadick, Coccimiglio, and Agosti piled into Hayes's car. It had been snowing in the mountains, ideal for tracking prey but not for driving. In good weather, the group from Force could have started out early on Tuesday; all were accustomed to dawn awakenings. But they couldn't take a chance on having icy roads delay them. There was too much at stake.

The trip began inauspiciously. Not a hotel room was to be had in Pittsburgh, where more than one hundred people were jammed into the lobby at the Roosevelt, waiting in vain for someone to check out. The story was the same at the Pittsburgher and the William Penn. Conventions had nothing to do with it, said a harried innkeeper. With gas rationing recently lifted, there were just "a helluva lot of people traveling," he said. Referrals were made to suburban hostelries, which also filled up.

Hayes and her passengers had to settle for accommodations in the city of Indiana, an hour outside of Pittsburgh. This put them scarcely past the midpoint of their trip, hardly justifying the trouble and expense of staying over. They'd already made one expensive mistake, and the hearing hadn't even started.

No one slept that night. The miners must have been yearning for the drafty houses in Force that they were going to describe for the city folks. Even dressed in their Sunday best, the self-described mountain men would be fish out of water. But as they drove into Pittsburgh the next morning, they were entering friendly territory. That was evident in the *Post-Gazette's* letters section, now enduring a torrent of abuse for printing a letter a few days earlier, which began as follows:

> Your paper simply must stop its present dangerous radicalism. The espousing of the case of the lady doctor and the miners in sewage-infested towns is a case in point. Don't you know that miners are not people, that they are supposed to be just a bit sub-human, not satisfied unless dirty, unshaven, uncontrolled, and on strike?[2]

This stab at humor generated a wave of protests not seen since Jonathan Swift proposed eating poor Irish children in his 1729 essay, "A Modest Proposal." Responses threatened to overwhelm the *Post-Gazette* mailroom until the offending writer wrote again, explaining the irony and apologizing.

Joan of Arc and her troops were entering the Steel City. No one could reproach them, or even pretend to.

Flashbulbs exploded as they entered the courtroom. All the cameras were pointed at Hayes. Women's legs sold papers in those days, and everyone vied for a head-to-toe shot of Hayes. She'd hoped to blend into the background behind the miners, but the photographers had other ideas. Ignoring the men completely, they aimed for her.

The skirt matched to her velvet jacket was patriotically short in compliance with wartime rationing. Unwittingly, she hiked it up above the knee while running the gauntlet of press cameras—actually running, with legs working and body bent forward. Her right hand, protruding from a wide fur muff, clutched long white gloves. With her left hand, she tried to shield her face, as if she'd been charged with a crime. The effort was not entirely successful: she couldn't hide a smile.

An Associated Press camera caught the image. Perhaps the smile was automatic. Hayes liked people and had a pleasant personality. But it could have revealed something deeper, a mixed reaction to her own unsought fame. The *Pittsburgh Press* was less successful, shooting Hayes from behind her as she stood. The flash pulled her head around, producing an image of her face that was barely recognizable. The legs showed, though, and that was paramount even in news photos of Margaret Truman, the president's daughter.

According to Ruth MacKay, a columnist for the *Chicago Tribune*, Hayes attended the hearing "looking for all the world like Tyrone Power's wife, Annabella."[3] Puzzling as that comparison was, given the difference in features, it was certainly flattering. Power was a matinee idol, and his French-born wife with a single name had a film and stage career of her own.

The leading lady was in the courthouse, and so were the villains. A photographer caught them on the steps. In a long coat and hat, Dickson looked directly into the camera, his eyes wide open and his mouth tense, suggesting fear and anxiety. Lambert, wearing eyeglasses and puffing on a cigarette, looked pugnacious. McBride was the most remarkable of the three, with his massive head and barrel-chested body. He held his fedora in his hand, revealing an abundance of dark hair. He does not look like a man about to turn sixty-three.

The receivership, the longest on record, was probably the first to be connected with the film star Tyrone Power. The morning testimony provided by Dickson and McBride had less relation to entertainment, consisting largely of statistics. There were, however, some startling revelations.

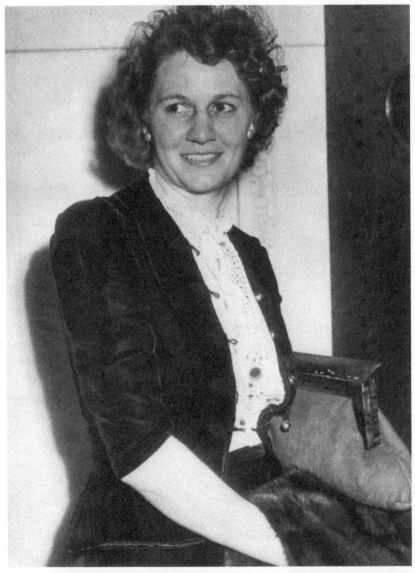

Dr. Betty Hayes prepares to testify about the Shawmut receivership in Pittsburgh federal court. *Reproduced with permission from the Historical Society of Pennsylvania*

As the hearing was called to order, Tony Coccimiglio submitted the miners' petition. Judge Bard accepted it and read it to the attorneys representing the holders of receiver's certificates. In addition to Bernard Goodman, representing two Pennsylvania clients, attorney Earl Reed was present on behalf of Baltimore and New York certificate holders. Bard accepted Reed's petition, allowing him to file a brief later. Certificates held by Reed's group had an approximate face value of $527,000, compared to $20,000 for Goodman's clients. Goodman, however, handled the questioning and provided the theatrics. His associate counsel, former Pennsylvania Attorney General Charles J. Margiotti, didn't speak.

The testimony began in call-and-response mode. Goodman read figures from the receiver's report and asked Dickson to verify them. As a magazine for investors noted, the surprise was that "no one had pressed an investigation before," considering the PS&N's performance during the war years "when any railroad worth its ballast was making money."[4] In 1944, revenues of $1,239,000 resulted in a net deficit of $256,000. Just the first nine months of 1945 had produced a loss of $220,000.

The strike was barely five months old, but Dickson ascribed all blame to it. "Our cash position is very poor, "he said. "We can't even pay a lot of our bills. Because of the stoppage we lost very heavily." As the miners had initially done, he avoided the word "strike." In court, as when opposing jobless benefits, he refused to recognize the action as a legitimate labor dispute.[5]

Digressing briefly to the sanitation issue, the judge said he'd received a letter from Dickson. In that letter, Dickson alleged that the state health department had declined his request for a report on conditions in the Shawmut-owned towns on the grounds that "somebody would like to get hold of this information." The judge asked the witness, "Is it true that this sentence was in a letter from the Department of Health?"

"Yes, your honor. It is true," said Dickson, who apparently wasn't asked to produce the evidence.[6] Assuming that he wasn't fabricating, the identity of the "somebody" eager to intercept state data isn't clear; however, the conspiracy-minded Dickson likely took this as further proof that dark forces lay behind Hayes and her accomplices.

The discussion returned to more earthbound matters as Goodman accused Dickson of speculating in certificates for his own benefit. Since his appointment as receiver, Dickson said he'd bought certificates with a face value of $27,000 for eighty cents on the dollar, which remained in his possession. He said he still owed a bank $6,000 for the purchase. More recently, without approval from any court, he'd used $47,000 in Shawmut

Mining Company funds to buy up additional certificates with a face value of $112,000 at a bargain rate.

When Goodman demanded an explanation, Dickson claimed to not have known that the Shawmut Mining Company was "technically" in receivership. He claimed to believe that the Shawmut coalfields were in receivership but that the mining company was not. Goodman responded by shoving a sheaf of court documents in front of Dickson and asking him to read them. All listed Shawmut Mining as one of the companies in receivership. Regarding the recent certificate purchase, the witness was foggy on the details. He said he'd bought them from "some estate," but he couldn't recall any names associated with it.[7]

The certificates had once promised 6 percent interest, which hadn't been paid since 1932. Now the holders of certificates had a first lien against the company. Dickson's latest report estimated the railroad's value at $7 million and the mining company at $3 million. Against this $10 million, there was a first lien of $2 million in outstanding receiver's certificates.

Goodman asked if the certificates could be purchased for ten or twelve cents on the dollar. "Near that," replied Dickson, adding, "Maybe more."

The judge interrupted to say, "I suppose the other securities are worthless."[8]

Dickson, had he been so inclined, could have said that securities had created problems for the company since its beginnings. In 1906, a Boston woman named Florence Cochran went to federal court in Buffalo, demanding the removal of the company's first receiver, Frank Sullivan Smith. She charged that Smith had diverted into his pocket much of a $16 million bond issue, intended to improve the railroad and make it profitable. Among his schemes, she alleged, was Smith's creation of a phony construction business that billed his company but did no work.

Representing the interests of numerous other bondholders, Cochran had been chosen to bring suit because she lived in Boston. The bondholders wanted the case brought before a federal court. They were wary of finding justice in a New York court: Frank Sullivan Smith, the Shawmut receiver, was married to the governor's sister. The suit failed after technical challenges arose, including the question of whether it was an interstate controversy. Smith kept his job until his death many years afterward.

Now another woman was facing another receiver, hoping for a different outcome. No one from Force had spoken yet. Bard had promised them the afternoon "when the more important matters are out of the way." But the morning was their creation, too. Their telegram to Washington, DC, had brought Dickson here, down from his throne. For Hayes and her three companions, it was their first glimpse of the receiver, who must have been sweating, however genteelly. To prepare, or to avert her eyes from curious onlookers, Hayes kept scribbling notes.

Continuing the cross-examination, Goodman asked why Dickson had failed to seek court approval before buying the entire capital stock of the Tyler Coal Company. Seized by the federal government in 1940 for nonpayment of coal and social security taxes, the firm was sold at auction. Despite Tyler Coal's problems—impending mortgage foreclosure and labor unrest—Dickson added it to Shawmut's portfolio. Goodman had been the attorney for the company under its previous owners. Very likely, that's why he knew of Dickson's unauthorized purchase.

The hearing also revealed new details of executive compensation. Ray Sprigle had previously reported that Dickson received $15,000 annually or $330,000 over his tenure. It was now learned that his billings for expenses were about $4,000 yearly. Dickson said this was mostly for trips to New York City, where he went "sometimes every two weeks or once every week or once every two weeks"[9] for sales transactions. Sales offices of other coal companies thrived in less elegant surroundings, without need to pay for a Lambs' Club membership.

Dickson testified that McBride drew $9,000 a year as assistant receiver, substantially less than the $12,000 Sprigle had initially reported. The *Post-Gazette* reporter corrected that figure and added some new ones. Several other Shawmut executives were pulling down handsome salaries for the era. Lambert, the general manager, made $7,200, while two auditors and a sales manager earned between $5,400 and $5,700 each.

Goodman asked Dickson, "Then, with all these highly paid assistants, who probably earn every cent they're paid, what do you do to earn your $15,000 a year?" Not leaving time for an answer, Goodman wrapped up his case. Reviewing the discoveries of Dickson's unauthorized actions, the attorney said that any one of them was sufficient to justify his removal. Calling the receiver a "poor businessman," the attorney ventured much further, suggesting that Dickson's speculation in his own receiver's securities for his personal account was "close to the borderline of criminal action."[10]

Next up was McBride, who testified that the Shawmut mines "almost always operated at a loss except during short periods and during World War I."[11] The railroad had fared no better, making money only in 1940 and 1941 over and above interest in certificates and depreciation. In an obvious attempt to undermine the strikers, he said the railroad made money only when the mines were operating. He said losses had been heavier than ever during the nearly five months of the strike. Suggesting that blame lay with the workers, McBride said he wasn't sure that Shawmut's coal mining operations could become profitable under any conditions.

Certainly, it would have been hard to make money as things stood. McBride testified that no new mine equipment had been purchased since Dickson was made receiver, and it was obsolete even then. This information followed *Business Week*'s revelations about the shabby state of the railroad, which had shed locomotives, coal cars, cabooses, and work cars since entering receivership in 1905. As McBride testified, the line had only sixteen locomotives. Some were leaking gaffers with only a few months' use left in them, and others had already been taken out of service. A one-time fleet of 1,635 coal cars had been decimated, and many of the remaining 110 weren't fit for long hauls.

McBride's testimony cleared up the mystery of how news outlets had gotten hold of this information. The general manager said that banks and other firms with a financial interest in Shawmut regularly received its monthly reports. Sprigle and others likely had sources inside these institutions.

The judge had a request. "Let me say now, that whatever happens, kindly in sending them out, send one to the court, too, will you?" said Bard to the delight of his audience.[12]

The afternoon belonged to the Force contingent. Betty Hayes took the stand first. Identifying her as "spiritual leader of the miner's revolt," a United Press report said she was "dainty" and "usually soft-spoken." That rather ethereal description may have been nothing more than gender stereotyping, or they may have reflected Hayes's ambivalence toward publicity.

She didn't try for tears and laughs, nor did she need to. As Sprigle wrote, she told the same story she'd shared with hundreds of correspondents, about leaking outhouses placed close to unprotected wells. She spoke of delivering a baby in sewage-splattered clothes after a fall into a ditch. Mud made the roads "impassable," she said, bogging down an ambulance and delaying her on her house calls. Human waste flowed through open channels, emptying into lawns, gardens, and streets where children played. Much of this had already been relayed through the newspapers. Now, however, the public was hearing it directly from the doctor.

At the time, home births and breastfeeding were associated with the unenlightened past. In her testimony, as always, Hayes was eager to associate herself with modernity. Leo Hayes, although educated in medicine much earlier, had also embraced these mid-century attitudes.

His daughter invoked his memory in her choice of pronoun. "We've taught our people to have their babies in the hospital and to care for them properly, using everything that science has taught us about baby care," she said, adding, "Then we have to mix our formulas with sewage and diluted urine."[13]

In this recounting of the familiar, there were a few unexpected twists. In the limited time allotted for testimony, Hayes complained that Shawmut had denied her a nurse to cover twenty-five miles of territory. That point was absent from the Pentz peace plan, but she seemed eager to impress it on the judge. Its inclusion suggested that her continued service was conditional on the assistance of a nurse. She also mentioned the $4,500 never paid to her father. As other creditors jockeyed for position, she didn't want her father's estate forgotten.

Testifying that the company had tried to replace her with "unlicensed practitioners," Hayes was not entirely truthful. By her own account, Shawmut had tried to thwart her plans to succeed her father by championing an osteopath. Although not an MD like Hayes, that person could have been licensed in Pennsylvania as a medical practitioner. As for Dr. Tonik, she could say what she wished. He'd fled to North Carolina.

The judge didn't press her on the licensing question. He also said he'd been following events in Force in the press. However, the Philadelphia and wire-service stories had been less thorough than the Pittsburgh papers, and one wrinkle in the story was new to him. Explaining how a suspected typhoid case had spurred her to action, Hayes paraphrased the advice she'd gotten from a state sanitary engineer: Why don't you wait for an epidemic?

The judge made sure he'd heard correctly. "You mean to say an official of the state health department said that." The doctor said, "Yes."[14]

For the second time that day, Bard seemed floored by the Pennsylvania Department of Health. To that old news, Hayes added a fresh complaint, declaring that some wells purportedly fixed by the company were still unsafe.

But the biggest surprise came near the end of Hayes's testimony. Speaking about the strike, she said she'd offered to "step out and permit an intermediary to settle differences," only to hear that Dickson was "too busy" to attend such a meeting.[15] That was almost certainly untrue. As Dickson's letters show, the strike started because of her insistence on inclusion and his flat refusal. She was the "outsider" who'd made a "mess" of things, according to UMWA official James Mark, who would have mediated without her if invited to do so.

It didn't seem like a mess now. For the first time, Dickson and his cronies had to account for their actions. Hayes's tenacity had brought things to this point; however, she also needed to hold on to the public's sympathy.

If she lied, as seems likely, she might have had gender expectations in mind. Spunky women might be tolerated, but obstinate ones crossed a line.

Tony Coccimiglio was the final witness, the only one of the miners to take the stand. For months he'd left the press interviews to Bill Agosti, perhaps considering the other man better spoken. In the courtroom, though, he was in his element. The director of the Kersey Eagles brass band warmed to his audience.

He began by asking Bard if he could be permitted to speak in "his language." By this, he didn't mean Italian. He'd sailed from Naples with his parents at age three and had been in Bennett's Valley ever since. Rather, he wanted to break the formality of the setting by speaking in his casual mountain idiom. As Coccimiglio doubtlessly anticipated, the judge gave him the go-ahead.

Asked to describe conditions in Force, he said, "The houses are nothing to brag about. You could swing a cat through the cracks in some of them."[16] Laughs erupted, and pens scribbled. The afternoon editions of the newspapers had a quote to set in boldface. Forgetting the hizzoners, Coccimiglio told Bard, "Come up some time, and be sure to stop in and get a smell of our drinking water when we boil it."

Now it was Bard's turn to stop the show. As it happened, he said, he'd already toured the mining villages in Elk and Clearfield Counties, "and I saw the back streets, too."[17] He also announced that he planned to return to the region, where he had relatives. They must have chauffeured him on his previous tour because now he asked Coccimiglio about bus and train schedules. He didn't disclose his impressions of the area. His task was to ask questions, not answer them.

Asked about the possibility that the men would return to work, Coccimiglio dropped the folksy act. Sticking close to the Pentz script, he said that wasn't likely "unless the company does something about sanitary conditions and a doctor which we choose."[18] Referring to management's refusal to negotiate, Coccimiglio skirted the issue of Hayes's participation, saying, "Dickson was too busy to take three hours off to talk to his own men." He added, "Today is the first time I ever saw Dickson."[19]

Bard ended the hearing by promising to hand down his decision by 2:00 p.m. on the following afternoon. Addressing the certificate holders' insistence on either a plan of reorganization or the sale of assets, the judge said he could not do in one month "what they failed to do in forty years." He commented, "It looks to me as if the financial condition is almost hopeless unless we attract new capital or squeeze out the water in these securities and get it down to an actual basis." For more details, the two groups of investors would need to tune in tomorrow. Bard's only on-the-spot decision concerned the mining villages: "The least we can do this minute is to advise tests of drinking water be made once a month."[20]

Advice was thin gruel for Hayes and her companions. They wanted Dickson's head.

The hearing ended in the late afternoon, and the Force contingent had to head home. The judge expected to announce his decision the next day. A Pittsburgh reporter, probably Chester Potter, promised to call Force as soon as he heard.

On the long drive home, no one talked much. Their confidence in government had been shaken more than once. They weren't sure how far Shawmut's influence extended or where Dickson had connections. McBride had left the courtroom grinning.

The Hayes contingent arranged to meet at the Force Hotel bar the following afternoon to await the call from Pittsburgh together. The hotel was on a party line shared with other telephone subscribers. One short ring followed by a long one signaled that the call was for the hotel.

There was time enough for food and drinks first. Almost everyone ordered a shot and a beer. Bill Davidson, the writer for *Salute*, called it the "Pennsylvania miner's drink." He was there, too. While the rest of the press corps awaited Bard's decision, he was with the people whose lives would be affected.[21]

There was another unfamiliar face in the bar room. Dr. Vincent Hayes had come in from Philadelphia to lend his sister emotional support. The no-trespass signs still hung in the vacant big doc's house. Vincent was barred from entering the house where he'd grown up. According to Davidson, Vincent was outraged. "Born and raised here for forty years, and not a place to lay my head," he said.

By now, everyone had consumed at least one drink. Frank Winkler had a suggestion for Hayes's brother: "Why don't you go and ask your neighbor for a bed?" Everyone laughed, knowing of David Bell's involvement in the raid of the doctor's office.

Some games of poker started to ease the wait. Betty Hayes went into the kitchen to help the proprietor's wife make more sandwiches. Everything stopped as a short ring was heard, followed by a long one.

Bill Agosti took the call. "Dickson's out," he yelled to the others. Their cheers carried over the lines back to Pittsburgh. Two new receivers had been appointed, and both were sympathetic to the miners' cause. They'd be up in Force within a few days to discuss things further and see about ending the strike as soon as possible.

More "Pennsylvania miner's drinks" passed over the bar. People danced and hugged each other. Miners swung Hayes around "as if she were a child," wrote Davidson, who noted each of the strike leader's gleeful reactions.

At age fifty, Frank Winkler was the eldest of the strike leaders and the most poetic. "Forty years of tyranny shot to hell," he reportedly said. "We'll have that Boston Tea Party now." Davidson continued:

> Betty started to cry. Vincent was sitting by himself in a corner. "I wish my dad was around," he said. Bill Agosti looked at them both thoughtfully for a moment. "Old Doc Hayes ain't dead," he said.

Her battle over, Hayes went deer hunting.

Some kinks had to be worked out, but it was a Cinderella ending. In making the announcement, Judge Bard had milked the moment for all it was worth, leaning back in his chair and wheeling slowly toward the waiting journalists before saying softly, "The court has decided to grant the prayer of the petition and to remove the present receiver."

Bard had chosen two respected Pennsylvanians to take Dickson's place. Thomas C. Buchanan of Beaver was an attorney and former state public utility commissioner. Robert C. Sproul, Jr. of Pittsburgh was a certified public accountant and an experienced receiver. Their first assignment would be to go to St. Marys "to see what can be done to open the mines at an early date," said the judge. The certificate holders would have to wait. As the *Post-Gazette* wrote, "It was the little group of striking miners, for five months just one skip from hunger and disease, who—with no help from anybody—hurled the 40-year-old Shawmut receivership into Federal court and made yesterday's decision possible."[22]

That wasn't quite accurate. The miners had considerable help from Ray Sprigle, who undoubtedly wrote those words for the unbylined piece. The phrase "no help from anybody" could have been a dig at John L. Lewis.

Again, Hayes's star rose in the firmament. Her photo ran on the *Philadelphia Inquirer*'s daily pictorial page, a kaleidoscope of images of the week's top newsmakers. "Fighter," read the large type under her face. She was pictured in the same montage with composer Irving Berlin and the international military tribunal trying war crimes in Nuremberg.[23]

The medical establishment also weighed in. Until now, news briefs in the *Medical World* and the *Medical Woman's Journal* had been her only recognition in professional journals. Now, close on the heels of Bard's decision, the Medical Society of the State of Pennsylvania announced its support. By unanimous resolution of the board of trustees, the society commended Hayes for "her untiring and unselfish efforts to make [her] community a better and healthier one." The commendation declared that a physician's primary duty was to guard public health, for which "pure and potable water and proper disposal of sewage" were essential.[24] However belated, the salute pleased Hayes immensely. In a state abounding with prominent practitioners and elite medical schools, the honor had gone to a country doctor.

The financial world also took note. "Dr. Betty Scores Victory in Railroad Feud," announced *Business Week* in the follow-up to its report on the ills of Dickson's receivership. This time it focused on the woman who had "started an avalanche" and had her premises padlocked in the process.[25]

McBride and Lambert would soon experience the sensation of finding strangers in their office. On the last day of November, a Friday, the new receivers arrived at PS&N headquarters with Judge Bard, who'd traveled icy roads to be with them. A meeting was scheduled with the miners' committee. The judge's presence was probably unnecessary, but for a keenly interested public, it underscored the importance of this event.

As it turned out, Bard didn't need to slog over to Force. The miners' committee came to St. Marys instead. Dropping their town-committee titles, Coccimiglio and the other Force activists represented their local. They were joined by John Challingsworth, the Hollywood local president. This was the same group that had met with management in early July. Then, they'd let the doctor take the lead before some of them, at least, privately arranged to return without her. Her threat to leave the area had quashed that second meeting, ensuring her participation ever since. Now that trust had been restored, Hayes was willing to be absent.

Two hours after the talks began, the strike was settled. The new receivers had pledged to do "everything within reason" to clean up the villages. They also indicated their willingness to sell the homes to the miners—"for what they're worth," one receiver remarked mordantly—and let the villages govern themselves. Nothing specific was said about Hayes's reinstatement, but it was announced that sweeping and repair of her office would begin immediately. The raid had left wreckage in its wake.

Both sides emerged satisfied. "We were very well pleased with the meeting," said receiver Sproul, the accountant. "We hope to turn Shawmut into a paying concern. The first job is to get coal mined and to get it to the railroad, which needs that supply—and that will begin next week."[26]

Actually, it would take a little longer. First, the rank-and-file members met at the Force church hall and voted to end the strike. Next, rock needed to be cleared from Proctor No. 1 and 2 mines. If this process recalled the premature cleaning of the Hollywood mine during the thwarted back-to-work movement, no one was so churlish as to mention it.

Still, within a week of the receivers' first visit to the area, excitement was in the air. Hayes had been officially reinstalled in her office, where renovations were still in progress. Bulldozers moved along the streets of Force, regrading them for paving. A study of the feasibility of laying three miles of pipe to bring in water was underway. In the meantime, all drinking water was being tested every two weeks, and a survey was assessing other sanitation and housing needs. "The miners and the new receivers seem to like each other," Pentz observed cheerfully, as miners searched their closets for work jackets.[27]

Many of the old clothes didn't fit. During the months of idleness, some men had gained as much as fifty pounds, not ideal for coal digging. Still, a first wave of miners grabbed picks and shovels on December 10 and headed for the pits. As they traveled four miles to the face on the "man train," Ray Sprigle was with them, ducking just in time as they entered a low tunnel and noting the sensation of burrowing under the mountain ranges. He watched the men work in rooms with ceiling heights of three-and-one-half feet, standing on their knees or rolled on their sides. The narrow seam made this "one of the most killing mine jobs in the soft coal field," Sprigle wrote.[28]

Only about 150 men dug on the first day, with the rest expected to be called back over the next two weeks. The first day yielded a scant 129 tons of coal, compared with the daily range of 1,050 to 1,150 tons produced in wartime. Both men and management said it would be a long time before they hit that mark again. The receivers had promised not only to clean up the towns but to put the mines, with their outdated and worn equipment, on a sound financial basis. Like the miners, they had a tough job ahead of them.

The Pittsburgh papers took a particular interest in "Bobby" Sproul, who'd played high school basketball for one of the star teams in the area. In the service, the new receiver had planned bombing operations and Mediterranean air transport. Then he was called home to audit U.S. Air Force contracts with major corporations. Estimating it would take six months before he and his coreceiver "know where we're heading," the Pittsburgh accountant said he planned to spend much of his time in St. Marys.[29] Those words would prove prophetic.

Anxiety gripped St. Marys, where the various Shawmut companies had hundreds of employees. For months, the city's newspaper had been quiet about the strike and the receivership. One day after Dickson's loss of receivership, the paper's editorial board finally rediscovered its voice, lamenting what it saw as Shawmut's public-relations missteps.

The city had been under a gag order, the paper revealed. After Sprigle's series about Shawmut appeared in mid-August, "Word came out of Wellsville, N.Y., to say nothing to the press," said the editorial. And there lay the problem, it argued: "The local company was depicted as an organization not interested in what might be termed 'human welfare,'" while in St. Marys, "we know different." Dispensing faint praise for the Shawmut companies as "stable" enterprises paying good wages "in most instances," the editorial admitted that unmuzzling employees might not have changed the outcome. Still, it said, the company "would have been shown in far different status had it permitted the press to carry something in their news column in their defense." The piece concluded, "Silence isn't always golden."[30]

A free press doesn't need to be "permitted" to print news. Intentionally or not, the editorial was revealing. Dickson had held the town in his grip, suppressing sales of the *Post-Gazette* and telling the *Daily Press* what to write.

A mystery was solved. While Hayes commanded worldwide attention, a paper based fourteen miles from Force had gone silent. So had Frank Lambert, whose Boston Tea Party remark had traveled worldwide. As the strike continued, not a peep was heard from the mine manager until he reappeared in the office raid. When FBI agents came to St. Marys, no one chronicled their movements around town. As Shawmut's balance sheets were discussed in national magazines, the *Daily Press* gathered no quotes from the company's legions of white-collar workers, not even anonymously.

On the other hand, the St. Marys paper wrote nothing to champion the company, condemn Hayes and the strikers, or decry the federal investigation. It had been more than willing to do so, the editorial suggested, but Dickson wanted it all kept mum "with the presumption, we suppose, the whole thing would blow over in due time. But it didn't blow over."[31]

Even if unhappy about its liberation, the *Daily Press* could now choose what to cover. As the receivers pondered the Shawmut Line's fate, the newspaper produced steady fodder for Randolph Soranson's scrapbook. Despite the ascent of the carbon industry, St. Marys was still a railroad town with tracks crossing its heart. Locals hoped for salvation from big players like the Pennsy, which ran trains here for interchange. There was also fear that the road could be abandoned, an unusual step requiring approval from the Interstate Commerce Commission. Dickson claimed to have considered ending rail service, although as he wrote to Mark, the union official, "One, of course, hears that the operation of a railroad cannot be abandoned."[32]

For the one thousand workers employed by the rail line between St. Marys and its terminus in New York State, rescue could have come from the Reconstruction Finance Authority. But that was not a realistic possibility, as the new receivers learned before accepting their post. Talking to them by phone before the receivership hearing, Judge Bard was told that the odds of their lending to Shawmut were "not very good."[33] According to one observer, this potential lifeline was severed by another railroad. The "other" Shawmut Line, the Pittsburg & Shawmut, had no interest in saving its former sibling. Holding many PS&N receiver's certificates, the P&S had a first lien on revenues that might result from sales of its namesake's assets. It didn't want a government lender to jump to the head of the line.

Such matters might have been resolved by the Interstate Commerce Commission or the U.S. Senate committee that oversaw it. After the committee chairman, Senator Wheeler, announced his intention to investigate other "scandalous" long-term railroad receiverships, news reports said that Wheeler and another committee member, Senator Clyde Reed of Kansas, would call Hayes as a witness. Reed issued a denial, stating that Hayes could come and testify if she wished, but she wouldn't be called. Mentioning her in its brief item about the Senate, the United Press reported that Senator Reed denied having invited the "attractive physician." The phrasing sounded almost lascivious.[34]

For most, that ended interest in the railroad. It had no direct connection to Hayes, and she was the story. However, at least one person was concerned about another player in the narrative. Allen wrote to Soranson, asking how Erich was doing as he faced possible criminal conviction. The rail historian hadn't forgotten his drive with the company cop to the Kasson Loop, cited in the long-ago bondholder's suit as a deplorable waste of money.

With his nebulous job title, new bosses, and legal troubles, Erich might have been facing an uncertain future. For the moment, though, his mind was on other things. Answering Charles Allen's query, Soranson wrote, "Mr. Erich is around every day, and he told me last Saturday that he had shot a large buck that day and seemed quite elated over the fact, but I have heard nothing further about the Shawmut incident from him or Mrs. Erich, who is in the store frequently." There would be no new developments in the case of the raid on the doctor's office until January, he added.[35]

Many of his fellow employees weren't so easily distracted. "Many heads will fall in the Shawmut offices," Soranson wrote, having gathered that this was the general consensus. Unraveling the long-standing mystery of why Shawmut employed so many clerks, the new receivers had found that "a monied racket for big pay has been going on for many years, with very little time spent in the offices." Instead, wrote the grocer, "Officials and clerks frequent lodge and club rooms a majority of the period which constitutes their day's labor."[36]

For the time being, Dickson, McBride, and Lambert remained at their posts. Presumably, the new management kept the latter two at their desks and away from the lodges. Out of leash range in Wellsville, Dickson wasn't going to give up easily. Still determined to punish the rebellious miners, he filed a second appeal of their jobless benefits. His former corporate attorney had announced plans for this last-ditch effort soon after Hayes was thrown out of her office. At that time, the company maintained that it had hired another physician who would soon begin work. Apparently, that final appeal had never been heard. Incredibly, Dickson managed to revive it after his dismissal. Like a dog with a bone, he just wouldn't quit.

Never mind that many of the miners were already back at work. The case was scheduled to be heard by the chairman of the Unemployment Compensation Board. This time it would go to the top, not to a regional referee. But the new receivers, through their attorneys, had the hearing continued to January. Expressing their support for the miners' unemployment benefits, they said they would ask Judge Bard for permission to withdraw the appeal.

Undeterred, Dickson refused to relinquish the Shawmut's New York properties to the new receivers, maintaining that he still had control of them through his appointment as receiver by a county court in that state. Indeed, he'd been appointed there, as well as in Pennsylvania, because the corporate properties straddled the states. It had all happened in a rush after the sudden death of his immediate predecessor. Henry R. Hastings had been receiver for barely three years when he collapsed in his son's room at Yale.

The first receiver, Frank Sullivan Smith, had also died unexpectedly although, in his case, after a long tenure. The company's next designate had youth in his favor. Dickson, thirty-three at the time, had a long receivership ahead of him. "Another Angelica boy has stepped into a position of distinction," reported a local newspaper, applauding young Dickson's plunge "into the limelight" and assumption of a responsibility "that will test his ability to manage." His father, Dawson D. Dickson, was Shawmut's attorney at the time.[37]

Sproul and Buchanan said they would petition the New York court to oust Dickson there. In the meantime, Wellsville buzzed with showers and bridge parties for Jane Dickson, who would be married there in a few weeks. A church ceremony was to be followed by a reception for 120 at the Dickson home, to be festooned with white flowers for the occasion. The younger Dickson daughter, Marilyn, would be maid of honor. In a sign of the changing times, Jane had quit her wartime job at a bank in Manhattan, and her fiancé had packed away his air medals to begin a career in sales.

As children, Jane and Marilyn had seen their names, combined into "Janelyn," on a showy observation car still owned by the Shawmut Line. In 1930, with the nation plunged into the Great Depression, Dickson bought a used Pullman and remodeled it as a business car. New carpets and drapes decorated its staterooms, lined in mahogany with olive-green ceilings. The exterior, too, was green to match the Shawmut Line logo. A telephone could be connected with the system at St. Marys. In this luxurious rolling office, Dickson used to entertain business customers, sometimes taking them on tours of mines.[38] In more recent years, the Janelyn had seen very little use. In 1942 it took army officers and Erie Railroad officials over the Shawmut route. They were exploring contingency plans in case the Erie was bombed or wrecked. Ultimately, it played almost no role in the war effort.

Now the Janelyn was sitting idle. Unsuitable for carrying coal, it was of no use to the new receivers, although its steel frame and exterior metal sheathing, painted to look like wood, probably enhanced its value as scrap metal. Such calculations preoccupied Sproul and Buchanan, who'd taken on Dickson's headaches. They were more sensitive to the agony and—at least for now—not as well paid to endure it. Bard had given each a monthly allowance of $675, woefully inadequate for a job that, as they soon discovered, was consuming all their time. As they looked into the cash drawer, the outlook darkened further. They couldn't keep things afloat, even for a few months, without borrowing more money.

As 1945 drew to a close, the *Pittsburgh Press* listed Hayes's resignation and Dickson's dismissal as two of the year's major news events. Its reporter, Chester Potter, once had questioned whether the doctor's demands were realistic, given Shawmut's financial woes. Now he was a convert, contributing a four-column illustrated feature about Hayes titled "Dr. Betty Fights for Her People" to the celebrities section of a St. Louis paper. Trumping them all, *Time* magazine summarized her victory in its section about medicine. A caption under her photo read, "She Wouldn't Wait for an Epidemic." The *Time* article ended with a quote from Judge Bard: "Pure water should be the first requirement of a community. I think it would pay in the end to clean up. It is economically wise to make a better community."[39]

It wasn't paying yet, though. Less than a month after their appointment, the new receivers asked Bard to let them borrow money. Otherwise, they said, they would need to shut the Shawmut mines and permit them to flood. The till was empty. The railroad had only $17,600 on hand. The mining company's cash drawer was nearly empty with $2,700.

Running seven trains a day, the railroad was generating a $6,400 monthly loss. The mines were doing somewhat better, averaging a $7,800 monthly profit. But it wasn't enough. Just to meet payroll, the receivers needed $168,000 every four weeks.

The receivers desperately needed $200,000 to fix the business or dispose of it. With banks wary and the Reconstruction Finance Authority balking, there was one solution: They would have to issue new receiver's certificates.

The judge gave them the nod. The loan would be secured by all the combined assets of the Shawmut companies. Engineers had estimated the value of the mines and the railroads at $5 million. One bright spot in all this came from the engineering survey, which found "huge unmined tonnage" in Shawmut's mines. In addition to the Proctor mines, this included the one at Brandy Camp and those owned by the Kersey Mining Company, another wholly-owned Shawmut subsidiary. According to the survey, nearly 50 million tons of coal had yet to be dug, enough to keep the mines operating for another half-century. So much for Lambert's rationale about letting the coal towns rot. According to him, the Shawmut mines were near the end of their useful lives.

In allowing Sproul and Buchanan to take on more debt, Bard dismissed the objections of the P&S Railroad, which, after blocking aid from the Reconstruction Finance Authority, had less luck with the judge. The "other" Shawmut, based in Kittanning, Pennsylvania, was behaving like an evil twin, trying to wring out some of the money due it from the PS&N, regardless of the consequences. Around this time, Soranson was delighted to receive a surprise visit from two officials of the Kittanning-based railroad. They came to the store, but it was a social visit. They remembered Soranson from his days as a private secretary to several railroads, including the PS&N in its early days. Eager to pass on information to Allen, Soranson plied them with questions about their purpose in coming to St. Marys.

"They did not dwell on the nature of their visit," Soranson wrote, but he persuaded them to confirm a newspaper article stating that the Kittanning-based Shawmut had invested three million dollars in one of the early issues of receiver's certificates, around 1915, which had accrued thousands of dollars in unpaid interest since. One of the grocer's visitors was an auditor, who said of the loan, "Surely it should have some priority considering the scope and elapsed time."[40]

Eventually, the Kittanning-based Shawmut made some sort of peace with the new receivers in St. Marys. The other railroad lent Sproul and Buchanan a specially modified Cadillac to show off their properties to potential buyers. A ride in the Cadillac fitted with train wheels made the right modern impression. No one these days would want to sit in the Janelyn behind a wheezing old locomotive.

The new year of 1946 began on an anxious note for the receivers, but Hayes and the miners of Bennett's Valley enjoyed a moment of respite. With national press attention focused elsewhere, Hayes was invited to speak at a Lions Club meeting in Oil City. It was the type of male-only lodge in which Shawmut officials had whiled away their workdays. Her speech, "The Story of a Mining Town," drew a record audience of seventy-two members and guests. A local paper described her as the central figure in "the only strike ever to be led by a woman."[41]

Force was still in dire need of improvement. Beyond describing the coal camp's water crisis and running sewage, Hayes also spoke of its lesser-known problems. Still insistent on the "blueprint" for change that had shocked Dickson into accepting her resignation, she wouldn't be satisfied until all its points were met. Broadening the definition of public health, she included the need for recreation, still limited in Force to crap games under the church steps. The death of thirteen-year-old Diana Volpe, struck while walking home from the Penfield picture show, had not been forgotten.

Less than ninety miles from Force, the Oil City Lion's Club might have been on another planet. Hayes told its members and guests of the isolation of the Bennett's Valley coal camps, produced by the nightly shutoff of telephone service and unspeakable road conditions. Speaking in January, she invited her attentive listeners to visit while warning that, at this time of year, it was a perilous drive. The event was such a hit that the city's Rotary club booked her for the following month.

First, the doctor had a court date with the men who'd dismantled her office. On January 14, District Attorney Edward Blatt convinced a grand jury in Ridgway to indict Lambert, Bell, and Erich on forcible entry into the office, forcible detainer—unlawfully occupying the premises—and conspiracy. Hayes had withdrawn her charges of burglary and larceny, probably on Blatt's advice. As Chester Potter had inconveniently pointed out in print, her property had been moved but made available to her.

At any rate, the company had already been found guilty of burglary where and when it mattered—in the court of public opinion before the receivership hearing. Even now, as the trial loomed, the current issue of a journal for a typesetters union described how Hayes found "great, big company men" in charge of her office. Describing the confiscation of her medicine, the piece ended with an outraged, "Yes, that happened in America."[42]

9

RESCUE TEAM

In the part of America known as Elk County, the judge in the office break-in case was Henry Hipple. Hipple had previously worked with Associate Judge Peter J. McBride, but new associate judges had been elected since then. The former Shawmut assistant receiver took no part in this one.

Commonwealth of Pennsylvania v. F. D. Lambert, David Bell, Sr., and Francis Erich began with jury selection at the county courthouse on a Tuesday morning. Twenty-seven prospective jurors were winnowed down to a panel of eight men and four women. Some were town dwellers, others lived in the countryside, and they ranged from youth to middle age.

At least three of the male jurors—Richard P. Zurfluh, Andrew Herzing, and William H. Davies—were newly returned from the service. Before enlistment, Zurfluh had been a clerk in a men's store, and Herzing had worked in a St. Marys shoe factory. Davies, who'd joined the navy in 1943, had served in Pearl Harbor and Iwo Jima. Another juror was tavern owner Clyde Birch, who lived among coal miners just outside of Byrnedale.

One of the women, Bertha Mague, had owned and operated a school bus company since before the war, driving forty-six miles every school day. In a sign of the times, she had just applied for permission to start a new route to transport workers to factories. Another juror, Barbara Wiesner, was a farm widow with five children.

Betty Hayes, the first witness called, testified about her regular payment of the monthly rent. She told how Erich had given a letter notifying her to vacate the premises at the end of the week. Yet on an afternoon of the same week, she'd found Erich standing at her front door and a moving van next to her porch. She spoke of discovering Lambert and Bell in the house while two movers heaped her furniture and medical equipment into the van. She repeated her conversation with Lambert about the removal of her belongings and her later encounter with the no-trespass signs and the padlocked door.

Parts of her testimony were corroborated by three witnesses who'd also testified before the grand jury. Tony Coccimiglio spoke of coming to the house while the moving was in progress to ask what was going on. He said Erich had told him that the doctor was being moved out and that he, as company cop, was there to ensure that no violence ensued.

Ida Parisi, a nurse for the school in Weedville, said she'd gone to see Hayes on a professional matter that afternoon but was stopped by the no-trespass signs. She said she'd observed Lambert and Bell moving around inside the house.

The final prosecution witness, Ann Dubish of Hollywood, spoke of entering the dark living room. When she switched on the light, she saw there was no furniture. Erich appeared and told her that the doctor had been moved out.

A welcome moment of levity came as the defense attorney, Thomas J. Gregory, cross-examined Hayes about her identification of the defendant David Bell, her longtime neighbor. Asked how long she'd known Bell, Hayes replied, "Since I was six years old."[1]

Gregory asked how many years ago that was. "Twenty-seven," Hayes said, smiling. There was laughter; many women of the era began lying about their age after turning thirty. Hayes's age—which had advanced one year since her fame began—had been widely reported as a badge of her youth. The defense attorney may have been trying to establish that Hayes, knowing Bell well, didn't fear he'd inflict harm on her. But the reporters present were more interested in the doctor's words than in the line of questioning.

The defense didn't call any witnesses. By late afternoon on Tuesday, all evidence had been presented. The jurors heard final arguments the next morning. Much of the case hinged on their perceptions of Hayes's state of mind.

The prosecution had sought to show that, although no violence occurred, there was a threat of it. Edward Blatt, the district attorney, asked Judge Hipple to charge the jury by saying, "The presence of five men and trespass notices posted on the premises constituted a show of force and threat of arrest, and if you find that it was sufficient to intimidate Dr. Hayes so as to prevent her from protecting her right of possession, then your verdict should be guilty."[2] The phrase "five men" included the movers as well as the defendants. Blatt also asked the judge to have the jurors consider whether Hayes's regular rent payments constituted an implied lease, which would have required thirty days' notice before Shawmut could take possession of the premises.

The defense attorney, however, emphasized that illegal evictions are a civil, not a criminal, matter. Gregory asked the court to make clear to the jurors that in this case, it was not the eviction itself that was potentially criminal, but rather how it was done.[3] He'd sought to establish that his clients hadn't made menacing gestures, issued threats, or done anything to instill fright or terror in Hayes. He emphasized that the only conversation between the doctor and the defendants was about where to deliver her belongings.[4]

As in all criminal proceedings, the prosecution had the greater burden of proof. Charging the jury, Judge Hipple concurred with the defense. He instructed the jurors that the charge of forcible entry required proof beyond a reasonable doubt that "there was such force used as would cause terror or apprehension on the part of the owner or tenant of the premises."[5]

The judge's instructions would have been no surprise to Hayes. In swearing out the charges, she'd said the men had entered her premises and detained them—in other words, occupied them—with "strong hands." The company goon, F. J. Erich, had been posted at the door for a reason. Many years would pass before security guards were derided as "mall cops." The feared Coal and Iron Police, including those who had famously bludgeoned a miner to death, were still fresh in the minds of many.

Hipple instructed the jury to deliver a verdict of not guilty on the count of conspiracy due to insufficient evidence. The judge's "directed verdict," as it was known, was uncontroversial. The conspiracy charge had spiced up the news, but the prosecution would have needed to produce documents or testimony proving that the men had schemed together beforehand. With that charge eliminated, the jurors had only to decide on forcible entry and forcible detention. Gregory, the defense attorney, requested directed verdicts on those charges, too—again, for lack of evidence. However, the judge entrusted the jury with those decisions.

Before the jury retired, Hipple observed that this was a case that had attracted considerable interest. Even if advised to disregard the press, some jurors may have found the attention stressful. Beginning deliberations after lunchtime, the jurors had a long day ahead of them. There must have been times when they were twelve angry men and women.

The foreman, Jerome R. Smith, returned to the courtroom twice. At 2:00 p.m., Smith, the owner of an automobile repair business, asked the court for further instructions. Reappearing an hour later, he declared that the jury was deadlocked. They were told to keep trying, and supper was sent in.[6] It's not possible to know whether one juror was holding out, or whether there were several. The point of contention never became public. With no transcript of the trial available, it's impossible to know how Hayes's testimony stood up to cross-examination. The only press reports mention her joke, suggesting that she wasn't rattled. As for whether she felt endangered, Hayes was widely regarded as a fearless woman. She'd stood up to a powerful company that had cowed men into submission. It may have been difficult for jurors to assess the situation by her reactions

After nearly nine hours of deliberation, the jury convicted all three defendants on forcible entry, carrying a maximum sentence of a $500 fine and one year's imprisonment. They were acquitted on forcible detention.

The verdict was returned at 8:00 p.m. on Wednesday. On Thursday morning, Judge Hipple delayed sentencing until he could consider whether the evidence supported the verdict. The defendants were free to go, and the jurors learned they might have wasted hours of their busy lives reaching a decision that could be overturned. The judge suspected this group of business owners and veterans of being a runaway jury, starstruck by Hayes's celebrity and incapable of making sound judgments.

The sentencing delay didn't make much difference in the press reports. "Found Guilty of Forcible Entry," read a typical headline, over a short item on a back page. The conviction was a coda to a story that had mostly concluded. Still, Hayes would be forever grateful to the district attorney. He'd helped her take the men to court when the world was watching.

Meanwhile, during McBride's last days at Shawmut, his name appeared in business notices of shareholder meetings for the various Shawmut subsidiaries. With rationing lifted, Soranson was busy at his store, but he managed to clip a newspaper column thick with these notices. January meetings were called for Shawmut Mining's various coal and mine subsidiaries, including the Tyler Coal Company, acquired by Dickson without court approval. There was also the Shawmut Realty Company, to which Hayes had faithfully paid her rent, and the Shawmut Commercial Company, which operated the company stores or "rob shops."

The supposed purpose of these meetings was to elect a president and board for each subsidiary. It's unclear how these elections could have proceeded this year while new receivers were weighing options for the parent railroad. In any case, the meetings had always been a charade. In a note attached to the clippings, Soranson wrote, "The directors are clerks in their accounting offices, who receive some voting stock to OK a pre-arranged director's meeting in company offices by the directing head." The former railroad employee added, "I have served in this capacity many times."[7]

That era came to a sudden end as a trio of saviors agreed to lease Shawmut Mining Company and its subsidiaries on terms acceptable to the new receivers. The seven-year lease guaranteed a minimum of $60,000 a year, with an option to purchase all capital stock within three years for nearly $1 million. The proposal, submitted to Judge Bard for his approval, also promised a square deal for the mining towns; it stated that a "substantial" portion of profits would go toward improving the miners' living conditions.

Pending court approval, the promises made by Sproul and Buchanan would be entrusted to three other men. The bidders, all from Greater Pittsburgh, were John A. Robertshaw, Colonel W. J. Stiteler, Jr., and Charles Denby. Of the three, Stiteler, as president of the Coal Operators Casualty Company, knew mining. Robertshaw was a famous name in thermostats, produced at the industrialist's plant outside of Pittsburgh; however, the name best known in social circles was Denby's. An avid supporter of orchestral music and a tireless fundraiser for Pittsburgh's Community Chest, the blue-blooded attorney had a keen interest in fulfilling Hayes's vision.

Born in China, where his father was a diplomat, Denby had served in World War I before graduating from Harvard Law School and clerking for Supreme Court Justice Oliver Wendell Holmes. The son-in-law of former U.S. Senator David Aiken Reed, a Pennsylvania Republican, Denby had represented the federal government on lend-lease missions during the war. While his interest in Shawmut Mining was financial, he was also aware of its importance to the mining communities.

Asked whether his investment group had a new company physician in mind, Denby said that he and his partners would "consult with Dr. Elizabeth Hayes and get the benefit of her advice."[8] As a *Post-Gazette* news piece noted, having "toppled a totalitarian receivership," the miners and the doctor could now seal their victory.[9]

Now that Jericho's walls had fallen, that Pittsburgh paper circulated freely in St. Marys. There, Soranson kept his correspondent abreast of reports about Shawmut, including his own exclusives. After what he called a "formal conversation" with a PS&N official, the grocer wrote to Allen with this breaking news: "I understand Gen. Supt. Bell, of the Shawmut Mining Co., has been discharged outright, and Gen. Mgr. Lambert is on the skids for early removal."[10]

His most startling revelation was about a secret operation involving the son of the general manager. "Lambert's son, who held a lucrative office position here, has also been discharged. 'Tis said he operated a mushroom garden in one of the plants," Soranson wrote. Mushrooms were growing somewhere on railroad property, perhaps in an abandoned freight car.

The son was J. Harry Lambert, a clerk for Shawmut Mining. The miners' lamps may have come in handy; they were commonly used in mushroom cultivation. Novel at the time and popular at New York steakhouses, white mushrooms often came by rail from Pennsylvania farms. There's no way to know if Lambert's son had made a go of it.

Lambert and Bell, convicted together in a criminal case still awaiting the judge's decision, were two middle-aged men, suddenly out of work. At sixty-one, Lambert was ten years older than Bell but better connected. Raised in St. Marys by a housewife and a tannery worker, Lambert started clerking for Shawmut Mining at age fifteen. While his son was growing mushrooms, Lambert had time to network at the local lodges. Even at his age, he might find opportunities. Bell, by contrast, was not a denizen of the clubs. He lived in Force among increasingly hostile neighbors.

On the last day of January, Bard held a federal court hearing on the bidders' proposal. It was clear that a lease guaranteeing a half-million dollars over seven years was preferable to the alternatives. A mining engineer testified that as salvage or through a forced sale, the properties would bring in $390,000 compared to their operating value of $944,000. Moreover, the receivers seemed eager to be rid of the mining company. Sproul said they'd already had to advance $68,530 to the coal subsidiary, taking the money from railroad funds.

Just as importantly, the three Western Pennsylvania men making the offer promised the mining communities a "square deal." In a statement that might have raised some cynical eyebrows, Denby said that, with "able management" and the "latest and best machinery," the prospective lessees hoped to increase productivity at less cost while enhancing safety and avoiding workforce reductions. "Nor do we expect to be the sole beneficiaries of increased efficiency and of the resulting profits," Denby continued, promising that his group "would consult with the miners and their union" about cost savings, safety measures and "improving the working and living conditions of the miners." As if anticipating disbelief, Denby added,

> Everyone knows that the coal mining business is an intensely competitive and risky one, but here we have good coal and not unfavorable natural conditions awaiting only the earnest endeavors of management and employees. We believe that with forthrightness and good spirit on our part and with the co-operation of the miners and their union, we can attain our objectives.[11]

It pleased the court. Bard authorized Denby and his partners to sign the lease. They'd incorporated as the New Shawmut Mining Company— "new not in name only," wrote a confident Sprigle. He began a report about the court decision by describing it as the start of "a new way of life" for "the men who dig the coal, the women who pack the dinner buckets, and the kids who lug the water from the outside pump."[12]

It would also be a new way of extracting coal. In making the offer, the New Shawmut officials had said they expected strip mining to account for 40 percent of their operation. An early AP report of the proposal had included that point, but it was absent from other coverage, including Sprigle's celebratory article. Ironically, the solution to Force's water crisis involved strip mining, a practice associated with environmental damage. Indeed, DuBois had recently fought a different company's strip-mining proposal, fearing it would contaminate the municipal water supply.

But New Shawmut delivered on many of its promises. A young army veteran, John Palowitch, replaced Bell as mine superintendent. Even with the new push for productivity, Palowitch earned praise from Coccimiglio, who remained president of the Force local. The new mine boss lived in St. Marys, where New Shawmut set up headquarters, but worked closely with the coal town committees. Coccimiglio said the new boss "was co-operating in every way possible"[13] as the village plans moved forward. The band-leading labor leader and the mine superintendent shared a common interest—Palowitch, too, was an enthusiastic amateur musician. At a meeting of coal operators and supervisory personnel, he played two violin solos.

Far from feeling complacent about all this bonhomie, Coccimiglio and his fellow strike leaders remained vigilant. They'd fought a hard battle against formidable opponents without the help of their union. Writing to the UMWA's international board, the officers of the Force and Hollywood locals recommended four resolutions for inclusion in the next contract, soon to be negotiated. Their letter started with a hint of reproach: "Much of our hardships and a five months' strike could have been avoided if we had had the attached principles in the contract between the union and the operator."[14]

Omitting that first sentence, the union printed the recommendations in the *United Mine Workers Journal*. The miners' telegram to John L. Lewis had drawn no response from the international president and empty promises from an international board member. But the union paper had covered the triumphs of Locals 97 and 6397, and it now devoted significant space to their contribution.

Except for the first resolution—about vacation pay—the recommendations focused on health. The Force and Byrnedale locals called for the miners' right to choose medical providers and the end of administrative fees for health coverage paid by paycheck deductions. Much of this aligned with Lewis's goals. In March, the union president began his first negotiations with the coal operators, determined to establish a health and welfare fund for the miners.

To show that current provisions for health and safety were inadequate, Lewis had ordered a study. It found that miners paid $60 million annually for high-priced but inadequate health care, over which they had no control. Also, thirteen coal-producing states had weak workers' compensation laws, leaving few protections for miners with injuries or illnesses caused by their jobs. Where workers' compensation programs did exist, company doctors often testified against the miners in disability cases. The UMWA officials who'd conducted the study spoke for five hours before the operators' negotiating committee, producing volumes of data and citing dozens of cases.

No such groundwork had been laid for the final resolution from Force and Hollywood, which proclaimed, "No company shall maintain company houses for use of its employees without safe and approved methods of sewage disposal nor without pure water." Yet the union did more than print the statement in its paper. When contract negotiations began, John L. Lewis would demonstrate that events in Force had made a strong impression on him.

In a preamble to the resolutions, the valley miners strove to couch the spirit of a workers' revolution in free-trade terms. It declared that the coal operators were making "constant efforts" to strengthen their power "over the free will of the employees," thus denying them "common decencies" and "proscrib[ing] the liberties of free trade and the right of selection inalienable to all citizens."[15] Those patriotic declarations, with their veiled endorsement of capitalism, were written in the chill of the Cold War. Governor Edward Martin, now a candidate for the U.S. Senate, warned his fellow Republicans about the rise of "strange doctrines" that could "menace freedom" and sow discontent, as they had in Europe.[16]

But nothing could stop the left from finding inspiration in Force's activism. A Communist Party–affiliated group told the story of the strike in a pamphlet arguing for a national health care program. Quoting Hayes and Coccimiglio, the booklet was printed by the International Workers Order, which operated medical clinics and provided affordable health insurance to tens of thousands of members. The IWO would soon land on the federal government's list of subversive organizations, leading to its demise.

The *Daily Worker* hadn't forgotten Force either. Continuing to investigate company-owned coal camps, the Communist paper ran a feature about Ronda, West Virginia, with its dilapidated housing, disgraceful privies, and questionable well water. The nearest doctor was twenty-five miles away. Neither Force nor Hayes was mentioned by name, but they lurked in the background. As usual, the *Daily Worker* couldn't resist a slap at John L. Lewis. Speaking of his proposal for a health and welfare fund "which his appointees would administer," the paper's Sunday magazine expressed doubt that any of the problems described in the article would be alleviated. "After all," wrote the reporter, "Lewis has been UMW president for 25 years without troubling about mining conditions, certainly without changing them much."[17]

Regarding free trade—a popular topic in postwar America—the article noted that the coal operators embraced it, yet they discouraged entrepreneurs from operating on their property. "The miners, according to the operators, are supposed to buy everything, from soda pop to living-room suites, at the company store."

That era was coming to an end on the properties leased by the New Shawmut Mining Company. A month after the agreement was signed, Soranson reported the accuracy of his heads-will-fall prophecy. "Many if not all of the Shawmut Mining Co. officials and office force have been let out . . . and the office space has reverted to the building's owners," the grocer told Allen. "McBride, assistant receiver is definitely out." So were Frank Lambert and his mushroom-growing son. "Oh, yes," Soranson continued, "[I] understand a firm from Brockway has taken charge of all Shawmut mining town stores."[18]

That last reference was to the Beadle Corporation, which already operated two stores in other mining areas and a department store in Brockway. One of the "rob shops" it took over for New Shawmut was the company store in Force, so repugnant to Local 97 that it had leased its union hall to an independent store to provide an alternative. Stores not controlled by Shawmut had thrown the miners a lifeline by extending credit during the strike.

No announcement was made of the hiring of a company doctor. Hayes continued to practice in Force, where the miners didn't need to await the establishment of a health and welfare fund. They'd already chosen their own doctor and had a system for paying her. Continuing her rounds of the fraternal organizations, Hayes was the speaker at a dinner organized by the Men's Club in Clarion, where her father had graduated from a teacher-training school before going into medicine.

Except for these speaking engagements, Hayes's life had mostly returned to normal. "The most prominent citizen of Bennett's Valley," as a local paper called her, had slipped off the national radar. But her name and cause remained in the popular consciousness. Interviewed about his long career, the pioneering surgeon William O'Neill Sherman said he'd once worked in mining towns where "conditions were the same, probably unpardonably worse, than those Dr. Betty Hayes described in her fight for sanitation." No longer an obscure country doctor, Hayes had earned the attention of the world-famous Dr. Sherman, credited for sparing thousands of limbs from amputation with his innovative surgical techniques. The surgeon and his interviewer knew that a mention of Hayes required no further explanation.[19]

Meanwhile, Force was preparing to shift from feudalism to democracy. In consultation with labor representatives, New Shawmut had developed a proposal to sell its houses to their occupants at nominal cost, under conditions designed to avoid speculators from profiting. The company would also donate additional acreage for community buildings and recreation grounds. As noted by the papers, the houses were small and "below average" in construction, but the miners planned to make improvements. The proposal was put to a vote at a community mass meeting, and things moved forward—slowly.

It was a Cinderella story, but Cinderella would still wear her rags for quite a while. The homes, some of them occupied by one family for three generations, were purchased at an average cost of $375. Legal snags arose, however, and months would pass before the buyers could take title to the houses. Amid those problems and a general scarcity of building materials, the houses and privies stayed as they were. Aside from a new porch here and a slap of paint there, the three coal towns were as dreary as ever.

Pure water and a new sewage system would also have to wait. Lambert's skepticism about the ease of piping in water from Penfield may have been well-founded. At any rate, it was quietly abandoned. Instead, drills were digging deep toward a new water source in Force and Hollywood. Plans to pump water into a hillside reservoir and pipe it back to houses could require tax assessments or a bank loan. Ross Pentz, still counsel for the miners, was exploring the possibility of incorporating the communities as a Pennsylvania borough or as housing corporations.

In the meantime, water was still hand-pumped from the old wells. Following Judge Bard's tongue-lashing at the receivership hearing, the state health department tested and chlorinated the wells regularly. Mining families continued to feed their babies with what they'd once called "chemically treated sewage water" while complicated plans for change inched forward.

As it turned out, the only immediate—and highly visible—improvement was paid out of Charles Denby's pocket. As suggested by the miners before Hayes's resignation and the strike, "red dog," a mining waste product, was used to pave the roads. Even so, the bill for grading and paving amounted to $3,000. When questions arose about whether New Shawmut would pay it, Denby wrote a personal check. "We'd have done it, but Mr. Denby beat us to it," said Hayes, not wishing Force to seem like a charity case. While everything else bogged down in red tape, the paved roads signaled New Shawmut's good intentions. They were also a symbol of the union members' victory. Labor and the new management were not always in perfect harmony, but a public airing of differences would benefit no one.

The streetscapes were still grander in St. Marys, but uncertainty hovered over the people employed by the Shawmut Line. Unable to make the railroad pay, the receivers were considering their next steps. "The office force, as well as shop men, are very jittery about reports of coming disposition of the road," Soranson told Allen, adding that F. J. Erich had spent part of March in the hospital. From what the grocer could gather, the cause was gastric and sinus trouble.[20] Around the time of the company cop's hospital admission, Judge Hipple was hearing arguments about whether to arrest judgment or call a new trial in the case of Erich and the other office raiders.

The trial got a fresh hearing as a new publication hit the stands. "A new magazine called *Salute* has quite an article about Dr. Betty Hayes of Force in its current issue," the *Daily Press* told the people of St. Marys.[21] Spring was in the air when Bill Davidson's feature appeared, illustrated with late-autumn photos of Force in all its slush-covered glory. Marketed to and written by veterans, the debut issue had a definite left slant. It criticized the army, championed labor, and clamored for veterans' benefits. Three writers would soon quit, complaining of the publication's Communist bent, and a new format would decorate the covers with lightly clad women.

The *Daily Press* also changed, albeit less drastically. Unhampered by the new receivers, the St. Marys paper closely followed developments concerning the PS&N Railroad. As rumors swirled about the Pennsylvania Railroad's purchase of the Shawmut Line, the *Daily Press* printed a news piece about the alleged acquisition before dismissing it as baseless in a scolding editorial. Out of conviction, or perhaps sour grapes, the St. Marys paper declared the match undesirable in any case. "We would hate to see some outside interests buy the Shawmut, for it could be that such a concern would raise hob with the local organization," the paper wrote, using a prissy expression for "create havoc."[22] In fact, the so-called local organization, headed by out-of-towners Sproul and Buchanan, likely would have welcomed a bid from the Pennsy. But tours taken in the borrowed Cadillac with train wheels produced no offers. If none materialized before a May 7 court date with Judge Bard, the receivers would seek authorization to abandon the line, pending the Interstate Commerce Commission's approval.

As the United Mine Workers negotiated a new contract, Lewis encountered fierce resistance to his proposal for a health and welfare fund. Coal operators complained of having to listen to "endless repetition" of irrelevant testimony about local conditions they could do nothing about. "We have gathered to make a national wage agreement and to assure the nation of its fuel supply," said Charles O'Neill, chair of the operators' negotiating committee. "We cannot discuss company doctors and hospitals." When he threatened to break off talks, Lewis thundered:

> If you could muster up the courage to leave, you will be back. Whom would you get to operate the mines? Who would patronize your company stores and your company doctors? . . . Surely you know nobody else would enter your mines. No other group of Americans would have the courage.[23]

A deadlock was reached, and 400,000 miners in twenty-six states went on strike. As talks continued, the Great John L. paid homage to Force, as he presented the operators with a three-point resolution on health and safety. Among its requirements was that "the operators would agree to prevent contamination of drinking water used by occupants of company-owned houses" while also removing "unsightly sanitary facilities" from outside the houses.[24]

O'Neill called the resolution "a gratuitous insult to the operators" and rejected it out of hand. Neither Lewis nor the spokesman for the operators referred to Force, but U.S. Senator Francis Myers later made the connection. On the floor of the Senate, Myers read a passage from a news article:

> Mr. O'Neill knows better. . . . His own district, the central Pennsylvania coal region, offers a prize example of the disgraceful conditions American coal miners are fighting to erase. We are speaking of the Shawmut Mining Co.'s ancient, crack-ridden shacks, leaky privies, and polluted wells. The company couldn't be bothered last summer when the 350

miners living in the coal camps at Force, Hollywood, and Byrnedale, Pa., demanded water that did not reek and taste of sewage.[25]

While stating that he "could hold no brief with Mr. Lewis," and his "magnetic personality," the Democratic senator had a message for his colleagues: "Remember, a strike is not always occasioned by merely one party to a controversy." He added, "I wonder how many Members of the Senate have ever been down in a coal mine. I wonder how many Members of the Senate have ever visited a mining town."[26]

The senator also spoke about company-owned Kenvir, Kentucky, where the "honey dipper" truck sloshed human leavings in all directions. Promoting his sanitation demands to the media and the public, Lewis publicized the letters he'd received about the stomach-turning conditions. Magnified in size, the letters appeared in full-page newspaper ads placed by Lewis's political action committee. The ads were illustrated with a crucifix, driving home a comparison of the miners' burdens to Christ's sufferings.

Kenvir was the new Force—but with important differences. A *Chicago Tribune* reporter went to Kentucky's Harlan County to investigate. There was no Dr. Elizabeth Hayes to greet him. Left to tour Kenvir on his own, he concluded,

> Investigations, and in some cases, confessions, have shown that the miners themselves are responsible in a large measure for the way they live. Few city folk earning what the miners do when they work—from sixty dollars to eighty dollars a week—would live in the dirt and squalor some coal workers and their families accept.[27]

Sympathy for workers was waning as unions unleashed pent-up demands. The strike wave hit St. Marys hard in late March as workers seeking hourly wage increases struck four carbon plants that collectively employed thousands. Perhaps fearing a downturn in grocery sales, Soranson described the turmoil in uncharacteristically choppy prose. "All the carbon companies in town are closed down and . . . property of pickets, throwing upwards of 3,000 employees out of work," he told Allen, adding, "On top of this is the coal struck [*sic*] . . . and every mine in the district closed down. The outlook here is very bad."[28]

The carbon workers were asking for an hourly wage increase of eighteen-and-one-half cents, a standard demand at the time. By the time Allen received Soranson's letter, one idled carbon plant had agreed to the raise, and talks had resumed at another. The *Daily Press* was more concerned about the cloud hanging over the railroad. Indeed, the once-silent newspaper tried to shake its readers awake.

"Is St. Marys interested in saving the Shawmut Railroad Company from passing out of the picture?" asked an editorial. If so, then why hadn't its residents matched the efforts underway in the New York towns of Wayland and Angelica? Having learned that those municipalities would argue against the road's dissolution at the upcoming federal hearing, the editorial writers scolded St. Marys for its relative apathy. Several unions representing the railroad workers were preparing petitions for the court, it said, but non-employees had so far been silent. "Cannot a move be instituted in town by civic and other organizations to be represented at the court hearing in Pittsburgh one week from today?" asked the paper on its front page. But it stopped short of demanding action from the town's elected leaders.[29]

St. Marys was crying out for its own Betty Hayes.

10

REVERBERATIONS

Attention hovered briefly over Elk County as Judge Hipple set aside the verdict that had convicted Lambert, Bell, and Erich of forcible entry. Citing insufficiency of evidence, Hipple sustained the motion for arrest of the judgment previously filed by the defense attorney. His opinion, referring to Hayes as the prosecutrix, stated that

> no effort was made by the Prosecutrix to interfere with or stop the men from removing the furniture, and nothing was said or done by any of the Defendants which indicated that any force or violence was used, or that there were any circumstances indicating any threats or force, or any conduct on the part of the Defendants to create fright or terror in the mind of the Prosecutrix.[1]

The opinion took no position on whether there were grounds or adequate notice for an eviction. It said, "Whether or not the taking of possession of the premises by Defendants was done in a legal manner, is not the question at issue. If a trespass had been committed by Defendants and damage resulted to Prosecutrix, she would have her remedy in a civil action." To constitute the offense, it said, "There must have been at least such acts of violence, threats, menaces, signs or gestures on the part of Defendants as would make the Prosecutrix believe that she would suffer personal injury or danger if she attempted to defend her possessions."[2]

Hipple also said the prosecution was under no obligation to prove actual violence, but "it was their duty to show that the conduct of Defendants in entering the building was such as would be calculated to alarm the most timid person," and they'd failed to do so. The opinion also cited legal precedent, including cases dating from previous historical eras.

Far from "the most timid person," Hayes had testified that she'd been alarmed, and the jurors had believed her. Other legal minds might agree with Hipple that this was a civil matter that never should have reached the jury. Yet it had, and twelve upstanding Elk County citizens had sacrificed a day to deliberations. For those wary of the company's undue influence, the verdict reversal was scarcely reassuring.

District Attorney Edward Blatt didn't appeal the decision. The men had been convicted in the minds of the public when it really mattered, a week before the ouster of Dickson and McBride. Headlines calling the accused men "robbers" and stories about Hayes's mad scramble to borrow medicine and equipment had re-energized a flagging story. By contrast, Hipple's reversal of the conviction made barely a ripple. A few papers, mostly within the state, reported it in brief.

Lambert would find a new position with a clay company that, ironically, made sewer pipes. Erich would join the police force in Clarion. With the days of the Coal and Iron Police receding farther into the past, there were few available vacancies for corporate snoops.

In St. Marys, the *Daily Press*'s rallying cry sparked a nascent save-the-Shawmut movement. On the eve of the federal hearing, some concerned citizens hastily called a meeting at the Knights of Columbus hall. The plan was to send delegates from St. Marys to the Pittsburgh federal courthouse. If there were any volunteers for this grueling eleventh-hour mission, they would have found it wasn't worth the trouble. Judge Bard allowed the receivers to seek the Interstate Commerce Commission's permission to abandon the railroad. Any protests from St. Marys would have to be directed to the ICC.

Hope still burned in some hearts there. At least St. Marys had fared better than the north end. The receivers had asked Bard to allow a suspension of operations in most of New York State, including Angelica and Wayland. There, most of the freight was agricultural, more costly to transport than coal. Also sought was immediate abandonment of a short stretch of track south of Hyde, Pennsylvania. The railroad unions fought these moves, but fifty miles of track were abandoned even before the ICC heard the case.

As New Shawmut Mining paved streets, drilled wells, and arranged house sales in Force, its railroad landlord faced possible extinction. Yet the mining concern's benevolent new operators didn't seem panicked. Testifying before Judge Bard at the hearing about the railroad's abandonment, Charles Denby said "economic facts" would force the coal company to seek another carrier as soon as the national coal strike ended. New Shawmut still supplied two-thirds of its lessor's business.

Even with the strike on, New Shawmut was extracting coal, according to Randolph Soranson. Concluding another long letter to railfan Charles Allen about the continuing "siege of strikes" in St. Marys and his own travails, including trouble with federal price-control authorities about his charges for corn, the grocer wrote,

> I also understood that although the miners have not worked the mines for several months, strip mining has been resorted to in the Byrnedale-Weedville-Hollywood district, the upper surface has been exposed by steam shovels and other earth-working equipment and there is now about one hundred tons available for shipment.[3]

The grocer seemed unaware that the miners' union and the operators had agreed to a two-week truce in the strike to fill urgent national needs. New Shawmut seemed determined to squeeze all possible value from its properties during the hiatus.

Not everyone in St. Marys shared Soranson's gloom. Striking a note of optimism, the *Daily Press* reported that there might still be hope for the railroad. An official of a track workers' union addressed a second community meeting. He told of an instance when public support had saved another railroad from extinction, under circumstances that initially seemed "just as dismal." A town official, the borough council president, agreed to temporarily oversee efforts to drum up support from business and fraternal organizations and circulate a petition. If not crowded, the meeting was at least "well attended," the paper reported; however, it warned that broader participation was needed lest the Shawmut Line become "just two streaks of rust."[4]

Firmer foundations were laid at a third meeting with the election of permanent officers. A local attorney became chair while representatives from labor and industry filled the other offices. The St. Marys plan committee made plans to meet with its north-end counterparts at some midway point. The hope was to work on a joint presentation for an ICC hearing scheduled to be held in Olean, New York, in late August. Even as the south-end organizers announced those plans, operations at the north end were suspended. As the PS&N continued to huff along one hundred miles of track, the St. Marys committee girded for battle.

Petitions supporting the line's salvation were sprinkled around the borough, with storekeepers urged to gather signatures. Closely following the Shawmut rescue efforts with scissors in hand, Soranson was more an observer than a participant. If a petition was kept on his counter, he failed to mention that as he wrote Allen:

> The latest on the Shawmut is they are removing most of their office forces and understood from the foremen of railroad shops that their entire crew, with the exception of four caretakers, would be relieved from duty today, and that notice had been posted last week to this effect. . . . There is no authentic information that any other road is interested although the towns along the line have some hopes as well as the employees who lose all rights and have asked for a hearing.[5]

Things seemed brighter underground. A few days before the truce in the strike was set to expire, President Truman placed the soft-coal mines under federal control, empowering his Secretary of the Interior, Julius A. Krug, to take charge of contract negotiations. The operators and the UMWA were deadlocked, but Truman said both sides recognized that further suspension of mining would result in "bankruptcy and ruin, and loss of markets to competing fuels."[6]

A week later, UMWA President John L. Lewis scored a stunning victory as the federal government granted all his major demands, including a health and welfare fund financed by the mining companies. The Lewis-Krug agreement also included a wage increase, vacation pay, and provisions for workers' compensation and occupational-disease benefits even in states where such coverage wasn't mandatory.

In a special triumph for Hayes and the miners of Bennett's Valley, the government agreed to make

> a comprehensive survey and study of the hospital and medical facilities, medical treatment, sanitary and housing conditions in the coal mining areas. The purpose of this survey will be to determine the character and scope of improvements which should be made to provide the mine workers of the nation with medical, housing and sanitary facilities conforming to recognized American standards.[7]

The survey would define the problems facing the medical program of the new UMWA Welfare and Retirement Fund. Lewis hadn't ignored the pleas made from Force "in the name of humanity" after all. With the survey mandated, three remote Pennsylvania villages had charted a path for others to follow. Other coal operators would find it harder to claim that outhouse seepage was none of their business and too vulgar to discuss. Under the terms of the contract, federal employees would visit thousands of houses in twenty-six states, interviewing families about roof leaks and sparking wires, photographing privies, and investigating drinking water.

Hayes, however, was given no role in the survey, despite her part in its creation. The navy's top brass took charge. Admiral Ben Moreell was deputy director of the Federal Coal Mines Administration. Moreell placed the medical survey in the hands of Rear Admiral Joel T. Boone. Bristling with medals and decorations, Boone had thirty-two years of service as a naval medical officer, including as physician to three presidents. He quickly assembled a team of medical and sanitation experts. Virtually all were naval officers. Boone said he was assisted by "certain civilian technical advisors," but not one named Dr. Elizabeth O. Hayes.

Gender discrimination was doubtlessly a factor. Also, Hayes was associated with labor, and the survey strived to appear neutral. Boone and his team took pains to visit "model coal camps" like the ones featured in industry-paid ads, as well as those reeking with sewage and garbage. The hope that was both labor and management would seriously consider recommendations that would arise from the survey. The advice would address mine conditions and hospital and medical services, as well as housing and sanitation.

It didn't take long for one of Boone's field teams to reach central Pennsylvania. In addition to a medical officer, each group had an engineer, a clerk, and a "welfare and recreation specialist." An acclaimed social-documentary photographer, Russell Lee, shot thousands of pictures in coalfields. About two hundred of Lee's photos illustrated a book-length report on the survey published the following year.[8] Some, like one of a miner sponging himself from a bucket, recall the news photos that had thrust Force onto the national stage.

Lee's photos were often printed in pairs to compare the worst of the mining villages with the best of them. An image of weed-choked shacks appeared over a vista of newly built houses with neatly clipped lawns. The *Pittsburgh Post-Gazette* had used the same side-by-side format, picturing McBride's St. Marys "mansion" beside a cluster of Force hovels. The caption: "Just a Study in Contrasts."[9]

The pairing approach wasn't unique, and the similarity could have been coincidental. Still, Hayes hovered like a ghostly presence over the Boone report, felt but never named. Speaking of "the sore spots, the decrepit houses, and the disease-breeding privies that were the despair of earnest reformers earlier in the present century,"[10] the report seemed to willfully ignore a more contemporary reformer, who was not only earnest but also effective. What's more, she was a member of Boone's profession.

Sexism likely played a role in excluding Hayes from participation, or even mention, in the survey. The report observed that mining had the "singular characteristic" of being an all-male occupation, but that was also true of Boone's core staff. Aside from two civilians—Lee, the photographer, and a public-relations writer named Allan Sherman—the investigators were naval officers. As Hayes knew from her attempt to enlist, naval commissions for women physicians were new and rare. In photographing families, Lee is said to have been assisted by his wife, Jean, a former journalist, who put the subjects at ease and wrote captions.[11] However, Jean Lee is not credited or acknowledged in the published report.

The Boone report presented a stark picture of health-threatening conditions in most of "Coalvale USA," its collective name for the communities studied. But its quest for evenhandedness laid some of the blame on mining families, saying, "Long years of control and paternalism have almost completely atrophied their sense of responsibility as citizens. They have slipped into the easy status of social wards."[12] Those words ignore obstacles discussed in other sections of the survey, including the need for tougher state health laws. Still, the very existence of the study honored Hayes and her allies.

No longer a poster child for health threats, Force was still at an in-between stage. There'd been legal entanglements involving the transfer of property, and then the strike. Now, a small conflict erupted between the two good-guy teams, the receivers overseeing the railroad and the group leasing the mines from them. The controversy involved fifty-one houses built near Elk County mines abandoned decades earlier. Not occupied—at least legally—the buildings could be razed and used for building materials, now in short supply everywhere. Hoping to spur home improvement in Force and its neighbors, New Shawmut Mining began arranging an auction. But as ads for the sale of junk houses appeared in papers, the receivers raised objections.

The receivers, Robert Sproul and Thomas Buchanan, had a different plan. Starved for cash as they awaited the ICC hearing, they wanted to sell all the houses to one bidder. But New Shawmut had promised the miners, as well as the court, not to allow speculation during the home buying process. Similarly, Denby and his New Shawmut partners wanted local people to have a chance to buy the vacant houses without dealing with a middleman. After a pause of a few months, the ads resumed in the summer. The guarantee of a "square deal" for the miners trumped the railroad's desperate financial needs. As a June payroll for the shrunken rail workforce approached, the new receivers were unable to meet it.

Hayes, too, was set to miss a deadline. She'd agreed to stay in Force for only one year after the start of the strike or until a suitable replacement for her could be found. But as the anniversary of her resignation neared, she made no preparations to leave. Still a leader in the Force cleanup—or reorganization, as it was now called—she addressed the community on Memorial Day. A parade led by Tony Coccimiglio's brass band ended at the monument erected a year earlier when one Force man had died in the service. Since then, two others had perished. Other names on the honor roll belonged to the people in the audience. One young man was rapidly emerging as a town leader.

Back from piloting multi-engine planes in Alaska and India, Raymond Nelson shared the podium with Hayes. A few years younger than the doctor, he'd lived in Force—where one of his brothers was a mine foreman—until leaving for college. Before serving as a major in the military, he'd taught in West Virginia and worked for the U.S. Department of Labor. Passionate about community involvement, Nelson would provide a welcome jolt of energy to the efforts in Force. Among those hearing his Memorial Day speech was his future wife, Margaret Pfaff, who'd served in the Pacific theater as a first lieutenant in the Army Nurse Corps. The two veterans would soon join the Hayes extended family; one of the Hayes sisters was engaged to a Nelson brother.

A dance at the church hall capped the Memorial Day commemorations in Force. The mood in St. Marys was less celebratory. News of the upcoming ICC hearing had aroused a brace of suitors interested in the Shawmut Line, as a whole or in pieces. Pulses quickened as representatives of H. E. Salzberg & Co. stayed for three days, scouring the books and riding the trains. The company sometimes operated short-line railroads, at least for a while, before salvaging them for parts; however, no deal emerged from the visit.

Buchanan and Sproul had inherited a pounding headache. When they'd accepted their receiver appointments, for a monthly allowance of $625 each, neither expected the job to consume all their time. In late June, they petitioned the court for a raise, saying that staving off creditors amid other pressing problems was a full-time task. Judge Bard increased their monthly pay to $1,000 each, retroactive to their appointment at the end of November. Their compensation finally matched Dickson's, although unlike him, they were tethered to St. Marys with a pared-down staff to assist them.

The glow once surrounding them was gone, however. The miners had transferred their affection, or at least their guarded trust, to New Shawmut Mining. As demonstrated by the housing auction incident, the interests of the railroad and its mining lessee didn't always coincide. Preparing to suspend operations, Sproul and Buchanan had become villains in the eyes of the rail workers. The cessation of operations at the north end saved costs, but galvanized their opponents. A coalition of New York towns, businesses, and investors was challenging the receivers' authority in that state. Within a month of getting their raises, Sproul and Buchanan were back in court to face these new attacks.

Judge Bard expanded the two men's authority by making them trustees of the railroad with power to manage its properties "wherever situated." A committee representing various interests along the Shawmut Line's north end proposed that New York State also be involved in the naming of a trustee. The committee represented towns and shippers, but was led by the Bank of Angelica, which held many receiver's certificates. Bard responded by pointing out that certificate holders "had said practically nothing all these years." Urging shippers to take a "long-range attitude" until shipping could again be assured, Bard still seemed hopeful about a sale.

Officially, Sproul and Buchanan were both trustees and receivers. Eventually, this would result in far more compensation for each of them, but the double title was awkward for the press, which often referred to them only by the latter term. The judge, however, was eager to shake off the stigma attached to it. "This receivership existed more than forty years," he told the bank-led committee. "I am not allowing it to continue much longer. I insist that the reorganization get going or [that] it be sold, one way or another."[13]

The most likely way, in Soranson's view, led to the junkyard. Writing to Allen in August, he seemed less upset by the strikes in St. Marys than he'd been a few months earlier. Now that the miners and carbon workers were back on the job, he was busy at the store, naming "increased trade" as his excuse for delays in responding to Allen's letters. Still, he was able to pass on a bit of railroad gossip:

> One worthy officer of one of the larger carbon companies told me the other evening that Mr. Buchanan, one of the receivers, stated frankly in his office the other day to some businessmen that neither he or Mr. Sproul, the other receiver, were practical railroad men but were more directly interested in mining and coal deals and favored dismantling the road to the highest bidder, but it was his candid opinion if the road was

purchased by other persons with a genuine practical operating man in charge it could be made to pay.[14]

Soranson also suggested that his correspondent attend the ICC hearing on the railroad's status, to be held in Olean, New York, more than a hundred miles from Allen's base in Rochester. It was a shorter distance from St. Marys, about sixty-five miles, where the grocer could have joined a contingent of save-the-Shawmut committee members who were making the journey. In his letters, he envisioned a future in which "General Electric or some other large company with many subsidiary interests in manufacturing"[15] would establish factories in all the large towns along the lines, shipping its goods and equipment on the Shawmut.

Soranson confined his ideas to his correspondence, clipping another rallying cry from the *Daily Press*, but not heeding it. An editorial urged readers to join a group of St. Marys residents as they traveled to Olean to unite with their northern counterparts. The aim, it said, was to ask the ICC to postpone any final decision on abandonment. A year before, the paper had studiously avoided any mention of Hayes's name. Now it was making up for lost time. The petition to the ICC followed "the much-publicized 'Dr. Betty Hayes's case,'" the editorial said, not blaming her for the impending doomsday but linking her name to it anyway.[16]

Several hundred people attended the hearing. Most were residents of New York's Allegany County, worried about a permanent loss of freight service. The Quaker State Oil Refining Co. said abandonment of the road would jeopardize an investment of several million dollars it had made at its Bolivar plant and a half million more invested in a Farmers Valley, Pennsylvania, facility. The Bank of Angelica added its voice.

Speaking for both receivers-turned-trustees, Sproul painted a dismal picture of mounting losses, overdue repairs, empty cash drawers, and lack of appeal. In 1945 the railroad lost $901,045, a record it might beat in 1946 with a loss of $466,960 in the first six months. Obligations, ignored by the previous receivers, had grown to staggering proportions, but almost nothing was in the cash reserve. Sproul told the ICC examiner presiding over the proceedings about the failure to meet payroll on June 1. There'd been fewer pay envelopes to fill since then, following sixty-five layoffs at the north end.

Repairs were a year behind. If undertaken, the cost for materials and labor would exceed $428,000—funds that were simply not available. It was hardly a surprise that few were pursuing this prize. Sproul said there'd been only one "inadequate" offer of $450,000, not enough to cover obligations and less than half the railroad's salvage value.

No ruling emerged from the Olean hearing. The purpose was to gather information, which was submitted to the ICC in Washington. The trustees were asked to furnish more details, while those against abandonment drew up petitions to submit to the commission. It would take months for the commission to decide whether to liquidate the line or order it to keep going.

The branch lines to the coalfields were still hauling coal. With six years to go on its lease of mine and coal lands, New Shawmut Mining at this point seemed unconcerned about the fate of its landlord. Eventually, Charles Denby and his partners would voice their concerns, but little had been heard from them so far. Like the oil company that shipped on the Shawmut, they'd made a hefty investment that would be jeopardized if the trains stopped running. Press attention to Hayes had given the New Shawmut miners a protective shield, but now her name had slipped from the headlines. Just in case the magic was wearing off, Denby and his friends quietly prepared their own bid.

And why shouldn't the concerned parties of St. Marys come up with an offer, too? That was the question posed by attorney George S. Rupprecht at the next meeting of the local committee. In attendance were some guests from across the state line, including the Bank of Angelica's president and representatives from Olean and Bolivar. Rupprecht floated the idea of organizing an offer by selling stock in the railroad to rail workers and businesses along the line. He said $250,000 could be raised this way, and twice that amount could be borrowed from large banks or the Reconstruction Finance Authority.

Rail workers were enthusiastic, but other attendees raised questions about the likelihood of a loan from the RFA, which had previously refused one, and the project didn't get off the ground. That was probably for the best. Not long after this meeting, Rupprecht would start entering into questionable financial dealings. For years to come, he would be respected as a financial wizard and civic leader. Relying on that reputation, he eventually ran a scheme that caused millions of dollars to vanish suddenly from St. Marys bank accounts. Hundreds of townspeople lost nest eggs and retirement savings, and Rupprecht was convicted and imprisoned.

While attention was fixed on the railroad, mining proceeded. An explosion at New Shawmut's Brandy Camp mine caused a serious injury. A miner had set two charges to detonate on a timer. When the second one failed to go off, he returned to investigate, severely damaging one eye when the explosive blew up in his face. A press report of the accident didn't mention Hayes, but the man was transferred from a St. Marys facility to DuBois's Maple Avenue Hospital, where she admitted patients. Square deal or not, the mines were dangerous places.

Hayes found time to take a vacation—a real one, not like the sudden trip to Kingston a year earlier. The DuBois paper announced her September trip to Bermuda in a single sentence. It was just one item among dozens of gossipy tidbits. No longer trailed by reporters, she had the privacy she prized. However, others were exploiting her retreat from the spotlight to erase her from history. That became evident as Pennsylvania state officials reacted to a preliminary release of the Boone report's findings.

An industry group convening in Pittsburgh learned of the "disgraceful and deplorable" sanitation conditions encountered in a coal town by one of the teams under Boone's direction. The speaker, Admiral Moreell, shared a report from a medical survey team, noting that the investigators were suffering from stomach ailments and diarrhea contracted in the mining communities, which they described as "worse than battle zones." Reading from the report, the admiral continued, "There is no first-class water supply or sewage disposal in the entire county. All sewage is dumped into all the streams in this area, and some of the towns obtain their water supply from these massive, contaminated, polluted 'bacteriological tubes.'"[17]

The resemblance to Force was unmistakeable, except that the water came from tainted streams instead of disease-breeding wells. But the coal town under discussion wasn't named, nor was any location given—not even the state. And no one was eager to claim it.

It could never happen in Pennsylvania. Or so top-ranking state officials declared, scarcely a year after the Force protest. Richard Maize, the state mines secretary, said federal coal mine officials were "astounded" during a recent survey by the excellent housing, sanitation, and operator-miner relations in the bituminous fields. "I don't know of a place in Pennsylvania as bad as the report says," Mr. Maize told the United Press. The state health secretary concurred. Dr. Harry E. Weest asserted that the report "was not referring to Pennsylvania."[18]

Such comments were disingenuous. Dickson viewed himself as a scapegoat for the many Pennsylvania mine operators who treated their tenants as he did. Weest's department, familiar with the sanitation in mining villages, had dismissed Hayes as an alarmist. Outrageous as they were, these official statements went unchallenged. Indeed, it would have taken some effort to counter them. The Boone report conscientiously avoided identifying the mining camps that it visited and photographed; "In no case was the Survey directed toward any particular mine or community," it stated in an introduction, but rather "it was concerned with the bituminous-coal industry as a whole."[19] It presented a dismal picture, but no individual or company was held accountable.

However, the Boone report often made distinctions by state, and Pennsylvania had nothing to be proud of. The report skewered the state for not requiring regular testing of water in mining camps. In one Pennsylvania coal community, investigators saw children drinking from hydrants fed by untreated river water despite signs telling them not to. Throughout the state's bituminous regions, "It was unusual to find restaurants inspected by properly trained personnel," the investigators wrote.[20]

The survey also concluded that Pennsylvania was one of four states— along with Kentucky, Virginia, and West Virginia—where "typhoid fever might occur in epidemic proportion" in the absence of inoculation; it also noted the high incidence of "summer diarrhea" in the coalfields of those states.[21] The finding was a stunning vindication of Hayes, harking back to the origins of her protest. A year earlier, she would have been asked to comment on the Moreell speech in Pittsburgh and the state officials' denials. Now her starlight shone only over one corner of the state, where some knew her mainly as a railroad destroyer.

With her family, Hayes marked a special occasion. Her sister Catherine returned to the area to marry Joseph Nelson. The best man was the groom's brother Ray, who was aiding the Force development project. A church ceremony in Brockway was followed by a dinner at the Pershing Hotel in DuBois. For the mother of the bride, Anna, it must have been a happy day after so many losses. The three daughters who lived nearby were there—Betty and Leola, as well as Aileen with her husband and children. Another married daughter, Helen, was absent, however.

Vincent, Anna Hayes's sole surviving son, had come from Philadelphia. He was gaining a brother-in-law, but losing a partner. Catherine gave up her share of their medical practice to join her husband in Seattle, where he worked in the electrical industry. She would spend the rest of her life in the West and Southwest, never losing touch with her family. Several members of the Agosti family were also at the wedding. On trips back to Pennsylvania, Catherine would visit Henry and Martha Agosti, who'd let Betty examine patients on their kitchen table.

Those days were over in Force, where two guests at Catherine Hayes Nelson's wedding were officers of New Shawmut Homes Inc. Raymond Nelson, secretary, and Elizabeth Hayes, treasurer, completed a slate headed by Anthony Coccimiglio, president. Incorporated as first-class, nonprofit corporations, Force and Byrnedale could levy assessments for water and sewage systems. Speaking in her new role, Betty Hayes pointed out that, in good times, miners averaged $200 in monthly income. "That's $20,000 a month that we have to spend right here in Force," she told a reporter, as the spotlight briefly swiveled back to Force.[22] The first anniversary of Force's liberation was near, and journalists were looking for a feel-good holiday story.

It was going to take a miracle to get there, or so it seemed at times. By mid–November, the media was predicting a browned-out Christmas. Another national coal strike loomed as John L. Lewis canceled his agreement with the federal government over the formula used to calculate wage hikes. As hundreds of thousands of miners prepared to leave the pits, the trustees of PS&N Railroad pleaded with New Shawmut to keep its mines open. In a letter sent from one office in St. Marys to another, trustee Thomas C. Buchanan warned the company's general superintendent, Jack Alexander, that without coal shipping fees, the beleaguered railroad might have to suspend operations immediately.

The miners walked out anyway, leaving eighty-seven cars full of coal on the sidings. An engine was sent to move them, perhaps the last coal train in a while. The trustees had just made a small deal to sell a tract of land in St. Marys to a power company for $18,000, but they were still losing an average of $10,000 a month. A paper recording the land sale asked about the future of the Shawmut Line. A spokesman said they planned to maintain limited service "with the hope that the strike will not be of long duration."[23]

It wasn't. The dimout lights mandated in half the nation brightened to full force on December 7. In typically dramatic fashion, Lewis ended the seventeen-day strike on the fifth anniversary of the attack on Pearl Harbor. That left plenty of time for the *Post-Gazette* to prepare an update on Force, steadily following Hayes's blueprint for progress.

Ray Sprigle and a photographer spent at least part of Christmas Day there, visiting homes that hadn't changed much. Almost exactly a year before, his paper had run a picture of the Klaibers, a Force family of eight, jammed around a dinner table with three neighbors' children. "Kids in Force are welcome at anybody's table, anytime," said a caption. This year, the paper ran a nearly identical picture of the same family. This time the caption told a different story: "Soon T. A. Klaiber will own his own home—'company house' no longer."[24] The household was one of eighty included in the Force housing corporation. Another twenty-five had formed Hollywood Homes Inc. Byrnedale, not yet incorporated, would be the largest with 125 stockholders.

Home improvements were still barely visible, but "nearly every family here has a little, or sizeable nest egg put away," Sprigle wrote, and "only scarcity of building materials is holding back a miniature building boom." Perhaps because it clouded the greeting–card–perfect picture, he neglected to mention that many of the almost–homeowners were still awaiting deeds to their property.[25]

Real strides were being made toward solving the water crisis. Deep drilling had tapped a subterranean river of pure mountain water. There still wasn't enough pipe to run water into the houses, but pumps and machinery were in place, and a DuBois bank had agreed to finance the project. For now, water was still hand–pumped from chlorinated wells and carried home in buckets. But a new system could be in place by spring, and as Hayes said, "We are doing it all ourselves, remember."

There wasn't a photo of her in the story. It was picked up by the AP and reprinted in big cities where people still remembered her. Trying to stay in the background, she told Sprigle, "All we needed was a stake in this country of ours. We've got it now in the shape of our homes."[26] Yet, despite her choice of pronouns, she wasn't truly part of the community. After her sister's wedding, all her loved ones had dispersed in different directions. Force wasn't a home for her.

The holidays ended with a thud in St. Marys as the ICC ruled that the entire PS&N Railroad could be abandoned except for three small segments at St. Marys, Olean, and Farmer's Valley. The objections raised in Olean had not persuaded the examiner who presided over the hearings. In a damning report he'd told the commission:

> A railroad such as the Shawmut, without funds to meet its operating needs, whose credit has become exhausted . . . and which must depend upon the collection of prepaid freight revenues from month to month . . . cannot be expected to continue operation indefinitely even though certain industries may be dependent upon its service.[27]

The ICC ruling reignited interest from buyers. A few weeks later, the rail–riding Cadillac was pressed into use again for a deep–pocketed visitor from Mt. Lebanon, a suburb of Pittsburgh. The list of properties available for purchase included 350 frame houses in Bennett's Valley. Although subject to the existing lease with New Shawmut Mining, the coal properties were for sale—including the houses. Sprigle's carefully worded Christmas message from Force had said the Klaibers would "soon" own their home.

Charles Denby and his partners were preparing an offer, but they could be outbid. The visitor from the Pittsburgh area was Harry W. Findley, a "coal operator on an extensive scale," as the *Daily Press* put it. He spent two days surveying the properties in the company of a PS&N auditor. Any offer would be subject to the approval of Judge Bard. Nevertheless, these were precarious days for the budding democracies in Force and its neighbors.

No hint of such worries dampened a magazine feature about Force's "awakening." *Grit*, a popular publication about rural life, checked in on the effects of a "young woman physician's ire" and its "atomic vigor that is radiating over a good portion of the nation." Yet the woman herself seemed to have vaporized, apparently declining to be photographed or interviewed for the lengthy piece. A montage of photos includes an exterior shot of the doc's house with her shingle hung from the porch. Apparently, *Grit* could get no closer, and all quotes are from Coccimiglio.

Open sewers remained, but children were no longer shot playing near them. They were pictured instead near Force's new central well, capable of producing ninety gallons of water a minute. The plan was to pump it to a hillside reservoir. Gravity would bring it down into the houses. Coccimiglio praised New Shawmut's directors and mine superintendent for aiding the effort toward indoor plumbing, but there still wasn't enough pipe. Plus, there was also that other stubborn obstacle.

"We are just waiting until we own our homes to really get things started—and it won't be long," added Coccimiglio, president of a housing corporation. The piece described the houses as company-owned, although most occupants had "signed up" with the corporation and would take ownership of the homes when they became "available."[28]

That depended on how Harry Findley's tour had gone.

11

FAREWELL TO THE VALLEY

Harry Findley had ended his tour smiling. The railroad's trustees liked his offer—$1.2 million for everything, including the mines. There was joy in St. Marys. The coal operator's interest had initially been confined to the mines. Findley had intended to operate only the coalfield portions of the railroad and junk the rest; however, the weekend visit had convinced him that he could keep the entire line in operation. An editorial in the *Daily Press* exulted, noting that the idea of keeping the railroad running "seemed as unattainable as man's flight to Mars," but "things seem to be perking up."[1]

Closer to earth, Findley asked the remaining railroad workers to waive existing wage agreements and "start with a clean slate," subject to collective bargaining. The industrialist addressed a meeting of the save-the-Shawmut committee, promising to pay a "standard wage." Office workers were so thrilled that, although not asked to do so, they also signed waivers. Leaders of the rail unions were more circumspect, taking copies of waivers, which, they were told, must be signed within days. Miners, employed by New Shawmut Mining, took no part in this lovefest.

Approving Buchanan and Sproul's request, Judge Bard set March 3, 1947, as the date for a hearing on all final offers. Advertising the auction, the trustees announced that they'd received an offer of $900,000 for the railroad and an additional $300,000 for the mining properties, including dwellings. The words "subject to existing lease" headed the description of the coal properties. Bids would be heard at the federal building in Pittsburgh.

Findley continued to demonstrate serious intent, meeting with shippers at a Pittsburgh hotel. A chemical plant and a clay company declared that they would have to shut down if the trains stopped running. There, the coal operator also met with representatives of the rail unions. They weren't as gung-ho about the waivers as the office workers were, but Findley stressed that he needed full cooperation to preserve jobs in St. Marys. He intended to operate the line on an experimental basis for six months or a year to see if he could make it pay.

Vultures circled in the meantime. On the eve of the hearing, the *Daily Press* rang a warning bell. "Rumors were rife today that several nationally known salvage companies may also attend this meeting to make offers for the company property on a purely salvage basis," said an editorial.[2] It ended with a call for concerned citizens to board a bus to the Pittsburgh hearing. Earlier hopes for mass protests had subsided: the bus capacity was thirty-seven.

According to the paper, "quite a few people" attended the auction in a crowded courtroom. Findley's offer was quickly topped in spirited bidding. New Shawmut Mining had formed a syndicate with a salvage company, Luria Brothers, to participate in bidding that drove the price skyward. A large Ohio scrap dealer offered $1,500,000 but would go no further. Findley asked to raise his bid to $1,505,000. He made clear that, at that price, he couldn't afford experimentation. Paying hundreds of thousands more than he'd intended, Findley no longer intended to operate the railroad. "The scrap dealers have bid us out the window," said Thompson Bradshaw, attorney for the Pittsburgh industrialist.[3]

A St. Marys attorney who'd served with Judge Bard on the state public utility commission asked to speak and was heard "with pleasure." Denis J. Driscoll, a former U.S. Representative, appealed to the court to keep the trains running "for the sake of St. Marys." He said that many employees had "grown old and gray" with the PS&N, never receiving a pay envelope from any other company. "What is to become of them, their families, their children—of St. Marys itself?" asked Driscoll, seventy-one, who'd been principal of the St. Marys schools when shoppers had bustled along Depot Street, and special trains took passengers to the Elk County Fair. Those days were long past and, as Judge Bard gently told the courtroom, "I am deeply sympathetic with the people of St. Marys and the employees of this company, but it must have been apparent that they were working on borrowed time for many years."[4] The gavel came down on Findley's second offer.

The forty-year-old receivership was over, and the railroad was finished, too. The Pennsylvania Railroad bought the three small track segments that the ICC had ordered to stay in business. All service on the rest of the line would suspend on March 31.

The St. Marys contingent went home feeling that promises made to them had been broken. George Rupprecht, the committee head, made his grievances known. Findley's attorney responded by suggesting that maybe if "someone from St. Marys, when the bidding was about to begin, had stood up and roared to high heaven and called all the people to bear witness, it might have done some good, but I doubt it."[5] Rupprecht, destined for infamy as the town swindler, was no Dr. Hayes. Suffering from a bad cold in Pittsburgh, he hadn't been able to speak at the hearing above a whisper.

The St. Marys paper wrote an obituary for its railroad with condolences to the affected employees and their families. The magazine *Railway Age* marked the passing of the PS&N in an exhaustive three-page discussion of its history and financial troubles.[6]

Others lavished praise on the trustees who ended the receivership. Judge Bard awarded them generous bonuses, each worth three times Dickson's salary. Betty Hayes was also recognized, in a less material way. "Credit for this goes first to a lady doctor who had enough gumption to stage a four-year fight for better conditions in the company's mining towns," said a *Pittsburgh Press* editorial. Perhaps because Hayes's name no longer sold papers, the editorial didn't even mention it.[7]

With the sale to Findley, Hayes's legacy could have quickly unraveled. The coal-town housing had changed hands. Again, Charles Denby came to the rescue, this time with new partners. A few days after purchasing the railroad, Findley sold his mining operations to its lessee, New Shawmut Mining. The sale price of $380,000 included hundreds of miners' houses. They would be "resold," Denby told the few papers that found this item worth printing. In Force, it made all the difference. The deeds were coming, and the housing corporations could begin self-governance.

Denby had stepped down to company vice president. Antonio J. Palumbo of St. Marys was the new chief stockholder and president. Palumbo, who often referred to himself as a "p.c.m." for "poor coal miner," had once dug on his knees. At twenty-one, he'd pooled resources with his father to buy the Underhill Mining Company, which owned coalfields in Clearfield County. Now, twenty years later, he was eager for expansion and saw potential in New Shawmut. The former miner would become an immensely wealthy businessman and philanthropist, with his name on college buildings all over central and western Pennsylvania.

Hayes would eventually see her hoped-for recreational facilities take shape, although not as she'd envisioned them. Two years after purchasing New Shawmut, Palumbo donated a tract of land to a camp operated by the Boy Scouts of America, on whose board he sat. A speaker at the presentation thanked him for benefiting the "future of boys in America." Ironically for Hayes, who'd fought for recreational facilities, the gift went to a group that excluded girls and women.

That was in keeping with the tenor of the times, observed the *The Worker* as it recognized Hayes "for her fight for sanitary conditions in mining camps" on International Women's Day.[8] One of a few dozen women so honored, Hayes was in good company. Other names listed beneath the headline "Orchids to Women" were Eleanor Roosevelt, former U.S. Secretary of Labor Frances Perkins, and civil rights advocate Mary McLeod Bethune. But this honor was only a sidebar to a less celebratory essay contending that American women were under attack.

The essay discussed a recent "flood" of books and magazine articles portraying the nation's women as "neurotics, incompetents, biologically inferior and a dangerous influence on society if they are permitted to enjoy equality in public affairs." Among the evidence cited were the magazine articles "What's Wrong With Women?" and "What's Wrong With American Mothers?" in *Colliers* and the *Saturday Evening Post*, respectively. A new book released by Harper Bros., *Modern Woman—A Lost Sex*, was said to echo Nazism in urging women to return to the hearth and childbearing.

The author of this analysis was Elizabeth Gurley Flynn, Hayes's longtime champion. "The 'back to the home' movement is on full tilt," wrote Flynn, observing that only a few years earlier, American women had been called "slackers" for not rushing out of the kitchen and into defense plants quickly enough. Now many of them, like Blacks and vets, were "sore, bewildered and shocked," she said, as "red-baiting, labor-baiting, anti-Semitism and theories of racial and male superiority are increasingly evident."[9]

Hayes, though, wasn't chased back into a domesticity she'd never inhabited. There's no way to know how she felt about the continued attention paid her by Flynn, chair of the women's commission of the Communist Party, if she was even aware of it. We do know that Hayes strenuously opposed the idea of a federally administered national health plan that would cover all Americans, or "socialized medicine," as it was branded by opponents striving to link it to communism.

In Kane, where she was now a sought-after speaker, Hayes made "strong arguments against socialized medicine," a local paper reported. Addressing a group at a Kiwanis club, she said her cleanup efforts "could not have been undertaken had she been practicing under a government-controlled policy." She asserted that "socialized medicine would stifle physicians' individual initiative" by swamping them in paperwork. She downplayed concerns about the many Americans who lacked health coverage.

"Many physicians generally care for the indigent under the present system" without expecting payment, she said.[10]

A hero to the left, Hayes was spouting the conservative positions of the American Medical Association, which had opposed nearly all proposals for a national health program. Indeed, national sentiment had recently turned against the idea. Less than eighteen months earlier, the International Workers Order had profiled Hayes in a pamphlet advocating passage of a Truman-supported bill for a government health program. Proponents argued that the program wouldn't threaten physicians' "freedom." Since then, a rising tide of conservatism had elected the first Republican-controlled Congress since 1932. The bill was pushed to the back burner, eclipsed by Cold War concerns and anti-labor fervor.

Tinges of those political changes colored the final version of the Boone report. The U.S. Department of the Interior released 13,000 copies of the report in April. With engaging writing, clearly presented statistics, and striking photographs, *A Medical Survey of the Bituminous-Coal Industry* was a riveting read. For those unwilling to tackle a 244-page report, a supplement titled "A Coal Miner and His Family" presented photos and stories in magazine format. Although filled with damning revelations about coal communities, particularly those owned by companies, the report laid blame equally on all parties involved:

> Management, Labor, and the families themselves are at fault for the inertia that characterizes the situation—Management because . . . it neglected, with notable exceptions, to fulfill the humanitarian obligations of its dual role of employer-governor; Labor, because its overpowering interest in . . . wages and hours seemingly blinds it to the importance of pressing with equal tenacity for housing and sanitary reforms; finally, the rank-and-file miner, because he tolerates eradicable evils.[11]

Blaming labor was ludicrous. The report wouldn't have been undertaken if the UMWA hadn't insisted on it. As for the "eradicable evils," the prolonged strike in Bennett's Valley, the attempt at drafting the union leaders, and the invasion of Hayes's office showed just how easy they were to eradicate. The Associated Press included that passage in its summary of the survey's main findings, although it was buried deep in a "discussion" section. The media, too, had lost sympathy with the labor movement.

Nevertheless, John L. Lewis reportedly ordered 25,000 additional copies of the report. Unruffled by criticism, he would have recognized the value of the survey. Supplementing anecdotes with hard data, it had found scores of other communities enduring the same hardships as Force. The survey would define the initial tasks facing the Welfare and Retirement Fund's medical program. And although Hayes isn't named in the report, the events in Force obviously inspired it.

In early June, Hayes announced her plans to move from the valley. She left her final destination mysterious, saying only that she'd first take a long vacation in Florida, "the first one since my graduation from medical school in 1936." There were rumors that she was about to be married. "They're kidding me a lot about that," she said, declining to elaborate. "She refuses to discuss her personal affairs," wrote a reporter, one of several covering a farewell ceremony.[12]

One thousand people gathered to say goodbye at Parker Dam State Park in the mountains above Bennett's Valley. A little rain couldn't stop them from honoring the woman who'd braved snowdrifts year after year to deliver their babies and treat their illnesses. Beer, soda, and popsicles supplemented picnic fare brought from home. Tony Coccimiglio's band provided entertainment. Charles Denby played toastmaster for a full roster of speakers that included District Attorney Edward Blatt. Three of the former strike leaders spoke "haltingly," said the *New York Times*, refocusing on Hayes after a long hiatus. Management was also well represented, as New Shawmut Mining president A. J. Palumbo joined Denby at the podium. But the honeymoon between the two sides appeared to be over.

Ross Pentz presented Hayes with a jeweled watch inscribed, "Dr. Betty—from the people of the valley." Her short acceptance speech included a final Rx for the miners: "Nobody ever cared about you before," she said. "Now you've got a group of men here who do care. Don't bog them down with petty arguments. Just remember that no mining town can progress with a company that is going broke."

Ray Sprigle was back, again participating in the events as well as covering them. Hayes's remarks showed her skills as an "up and coming labor relations expert," he wrote. Her biggest thrill of the day came when dozens of deeds were distributed to homeowners, he added. Hundreds more were expected very soon.[13]

Later that week, Hayes went to DuBois to accept a Woman of the Year award from the local chapter of the Federation of Business and Professional Women. She thanked Pentz, Sprigle, Denby, and New Shawmut official Jack Alexander for making real the "ideal of a better life among the mining people."

With that, she was gone, never again to become a national figure. "Life is looking up in Bennett's Valley," wrote the *Daily Worker*, observing that her departure had not been timed to the release of the Boone report but that the "one-man strike" staged by Hayes "had plenty to do with that report." Having "built a fire under both the Department of the Interior and John L. Lewis," the piece continued, "Dr. Betty has gone away, her work done."[14]

That was finally true when the remaining deeds arrived. As the *Pittsburgh Sun-Telegraph* accurately calculated, it had been a "bitter two-year struggle."[15]

EPILOGUE

Betty Hayes did get married, to a man named Charles Williamson. Her niece, Nancy Huffman, remembered "Willie," as "very hospitable, very nice" when she and her sister visited the couple in North Carolina, where Hayes—now Dr. Elizabeth Hayes Williamson—was a civilian physician at the Cherry Point Marine Base.[1] Caring for the families who lived on the base, she was still essentially a company doctor. The coastal area, so different from her native Alleghenies, enchanted her.

However, six years after her farewell picnic, Hayes moved back to the hills of Pennsylvania. She went to Brockway, still home to her mother and Aileen's family, temporarily taking over another physician's practice while he underwent medical treatment. A local paper said her husband was on active military duty in Korea. The marriage ended in divorce. Huffman wasn't sure of the reasons, but "I know he was a lot younger than she was," she said.

Leading a quiet life, Hayes—as we'll continue to call her—no longer carried the burden of carrying on her father's legacy. Her brother Vincent had divorced and moved back to the area from Philadelphia. He started a medical practice in Weedville and immersed himself in civic affairs. Grabbing the baton from Betty, he locked into battle with the local telephone company, arguing that its inadequate service endangered the public's health and safety.

"The spunky folk of Bennett's Valley are on the move again," wrote the *Courier-Express*, describing the latest "cry for relief" from the "backwoods." Vincent told the DuBois paper, "My father spent his life fighting power and coal companies. Now I don't want to spend mine fighting with a telephone company."[2] His comrade-in-arms was Denis Driscoll, the

171

former Public Utilities Commission chair who'd pleaded with Judge Bard not to let the PS&N Railroad die.

No trace of the railroad remained in St. Marys, not even the "two streaks of rust" once presaged by the local paper. Everything had gone to the recyclers, and Dickson's mahogany-lined luxury car, the Janelyn, was later spotted on the rails in Mexico. However, at least one newer business was expanding in the National Bank Building of St. Marys. A. J. Palumbo's sales and marketing subsidiary, Shawmut Coal Co., continued to sell coal produced at the New Shawmut mines while also taking over another big coal-sales operation. A Clearfield, Pennsylvania, paper called the move "added insurance for the future economic well-being of Bennett's Valley."[3] Labor relations hadn't always been harmonious, however. One conflict revolved around New Shawmut's lease of a strip mine to a nonunion contractor.

Taking no part in that, Hayes saved her activism for her personal life. For a time, it continued uneventfully. When her Brockway medical partner resumed work, she split office hours with him. At least for a time, she also arranged with a practice in Williamsport to see patients there. Then, hearing tragic news about the man she'd loved in her college years, she took the bold step of contacting him.

It was a horrible suburban accident, the postwar dream turned nightmare. A car crash in Maryland's Montgomery County killed Eleanor Lathers Voris, whom LeRoy Voris had married after his romantic relationship with Hayes. She died helping two sons deliver newspapers on a route in their country club community. The boys weren't injured in the collision. A third son, who usually delivered the papers, was at baseball practice. Dead at forty-one, Eleanor had left college teaching and a wartime job to devote herself to her family. She was an accomplished musician. Her eldest son, Larry, remembered the grand piano in their home on Manor Club Estates near Rockville, Maryland.

Aaron LeRoy Voris—he never used his first name—was working in Washington, DC, as executive secretary of the Food and Nutrition Board of the National Research Council. Sometime after his wife's death, Hayes located him and established contact. It wasn't an easy time for the family. Larry, sixteen when his mother died, said Eleanor had been the family disciplinarian. He said he'd subsequently been a "dumb teenager," making poor choices that angered his father. The one bright outcome of the tragedy, he said, was the "nice love story" of Hayes and his father. "I remember him saying, 'An old girlfriend who heard that your mother died has gotten in touch with me,'" said Larry, who described Hayes as the "instigator."

He said she was more obviously excited about rekindling the relationship than his "stoical," nondemonstrative father. Still, LeRoy was "very happy about it," his son remembered.[4]

On December 15, 1957, the couple married in Cherry Point, near Hayes's beloved North Carolina shore. The groom was fifty and the bride, forty-four. Hayes wore a blue suit with pink accessories for the civil ceremony, at which a small group of family and friends were present. The couple returned to the Maryland enclave where LeRoy and his first wife had raised their family. But Hayes didn't like it there, so they moved to nearby Bethesda. By then, Larry was in the army, and he would later settle in California, seldom seeing Hayes and his father. But it was clear that their marriage was happy, he recalled.

Hayes had practiced medicine in Brockway up to the date of her wedding. After that, she stopped working. Elizabeth Hayes Voris was LeRoy Voris's wife, "and that was her job," said her stepson. Returning to Brockway in 1960 for her mother's eighty-fifth birthday, Hayes showed slides from her trip to Chile, where LeRoy had been sent on a government mission to study that country's food and nutritional needs, and she had accompanied him. Now he was the one quoted by newspapers, as when he spoke about astronauts' dietary needs at a 1967 scientific conference. He caused a splash in 1969 by advising Americans to use cast-iron utensils, saying, "While you gradually eat away the frying pan along with the bacon and eggs, your nutrition will probably improve."[5]

On Hayes's recommendation, the couple moved to a North Carolina island community after LeRoy's retirement. They moved to Pine Knoll Shores, just west of Atlantic Beach. In 1976, LeRoy told a scientific newsletter about the experimental grass they'd planted to prevent shoreline erosion. "The grass seems to be doing fine, and we enjoy the big white herons that come in. There have been a lot more birds since the grass was planted," he said.[6]

Betty Hayes had come a long way from Force. "It was just a really fabulous place," spreading over an acre with water on two sides, Larry recalled. A state medical directory included a listing for Hayes at that location, under her maiden name. She was still licensed to practice in North Carolina.

Elizabeth Omega Hayes Voris died of a stroke on June 26, 1984. She was seventy-two. LeRoy believed that stress had brought it on. "There had been some problem with the neighbors there in Pine Knoll Shores, and he blamed that situation," his son remembered. Hayes's famous anger had spurred her to action, but it ultimately hastened her death.

Her body was cremated, and there were no obituaries, although the *Courier-Express* in DuBois ran two long pieces about her accomplishments. In 2010, the Mt. Zion Historical Society erected an explanatory plaque about her in a small park in Elk County, dedicating it on Memorial Day. That probably would have pleased Hayes, who had officiated at similar ceremonies.

On that and other matters, we're left to speculate. In life, she'd saved "everything," according to her stepson. Her sudden death left her husband with mounds of unorganized papers and letters. Helping his father dispose of it all, Larry and a brother found many unopened birthday greetings. "There were maybe a hundred bucks of ten-dollar bills that she'd never taken out of the cards," he said. Lining the length of the front yard with trash bags, they put it out for garbage collection.[7]

There aren't many traces of the past in Force, now part of Jay Township, either. The houses—remodeled, expanded, clad in siding, and equipped with indoor plumbing—have survived into the twenty-first century without looking like period pieces. Few would suspect them of having historical significance. That is the final tribute to Hayes and her allies.

NOTES

A NOTE ABOUT THE NOTES

Abbreviations

CFHA	Charles Francis Hitchcock Allen
IUP	Indiana University of Pennsylvania
JDD	John Dawson Dickson
JM	James Mark
PS&N Papers	Pittsburg, Shawmut and Northern Papers, Division of Rare and Manuscript Collections, Cornell University
RS	Randolph Soranson
UMWA	United Mine Workers of America

PROLOGUE

1. Julia Shawell, "Woman Dr. Leaving; It's Okay with Coal Co.," *Philadelphia Record*, August 2, 1945.

2. Walter Lowenfels, "Dr. 'Betty,'" *Daily Worker*, August 26, 1945.

3. Editorial, "An Indignant Physician Prescribes for All of Us," *Philadelphia Record*, August 3, 1945.

4. Judy Shepard, "Striking Miners Refuse to Betray 'Dr. Betty,'" *New York Post*, August 2, 1945.

5. Hilton Wick, "Doctors Are Funny Folks, Shouts Wick," *Leader-Vindicator* (Bethlehem, PA), August 8, 1945.

6. Letter from JDD to JM, September 7, 1945, Manuscript Group 52: UMWA District 2, Box 61, Folder 5, and Box 68, Folder 1, Special Collections and University Archives, IUP.

CHAPTER 1: THE INHERITANCE

1. Bill Davidson, "Dr. Betty," *Salute* 1, no. 1 (April 1946), 8.

2. "Bit by Rattlesnake," *Brockway* (PA) *Record*, July 29, 1932.

3. Nancy Huffman, telephone interview with the author, June 27, 2019.

4. "3 Graduates to Intern at Nesbitt," *Evening News* (Wilkes-Barre, PA), June 24, 1937.

5. Mary Roth Walsh, *"Doctors Wanted: No Women Need Apply": Sexual Barriers in the Medical Profession, 1835–1975* (New Haven, CT: Yale University Press, 1977), 224.

6. Larry Voris, telephone interview with the author, January 25, 2019.

7. News item, *Courier-Express* (DuBois, PA), August 23, 1938.

8. Janet A. Tighe, "Defying All Predictions: A History of the Temple University School of Medicine 1901–1980" (unpublished manuscript, 1988), chapter 3, 23–24.

9. *The Skull* (Temple University School of Medicine yearbook, 1925), 48.

10. "Physician to Go to Newfoundland," *Wilkes-Barre* (PA) *Record*, August 27, 1942.

CHAPTER 2: NO ESCAPE

1. Bill Davidson, "Dr. Betty," *Salute* 1, no. 1 (April 1946), 8.

2. Davidson, "Dr. Betty," 46.

3. Editorial, "Paralyzing Strike," *Courier-Express* (DuBois, PA), May 3, 1943.

4. Nancy Huffman, telephone interview with the author, June 27, 2019.

5. Davidson, "Dr. Betty," 46.

6. Associated Press, "Approves Women as Service Doctors," *New York Times*, April 18, 1943.

7. "Doctor Assigned to Dushore by U.S. Government," *Wilkes-Barre* (PA) *Times Leader*, May 11, 1943.

8. Katherine Scarborough, "Dr. Betty's Own Strike Still Ties Up Mines," *Baltimore Sun*, September 9, 1945.

9. Ray Sprigle, "Disease Stalks Company Villages," *Pittsburgh Post-Gazette*, August 17, 1945.

10. "Inhuman Conditions in Mine Towns Leave Coal Barons Cold," *Daily Worker*, August 4, 1945.

11. Letter from JDD to JM, July 25, 1945, Manuscript Group 52: UMWA District 2, Box 61, Folder 5 and Box 68, Folder 1, Special Collections and University Archives, IUP.

12. Editorial, "A Rural Slum," *Pittsburgh Post-Gazette*, August 10, 1945.

13. JDD to JM, July 25, 1945.

14. JDD to JM, July 25, 1945.

CHAPTER 3: THE ULTIMATUM

1. Ray Sprigle, "Company Financing Smells of Slums," *Pittsburgh Post-Gazette*, August 18, 1945.

2. Letter from JDD to JM, July 25, 1945, Manuscript Group 52: UMWA District 2, Box 61, Folder 5 and Box 68, Folder 1, Special Collections and University Archives, IUP.

3. JDD to JM, July 25, 1945.

4. Bill Davidson, "Dr. Betty," *Salute* 1, no. 1 (April 1946), 46.

5. JDD to JM, July 25, 1945.

6. Katherine Scarborough, "Dr. Betty's Own Strike Still Ties Up Mines," *Baltimore Sun*, September 9, 1945.

7. JDD to JM, July 25, 1945.

8. Ray Sprigle, "Disease Stalks Company Villages," *Pittsburgh Post-Gazette*, August 17, 1945.

9. All Dickson quotes that follow are from the letter from JDD to JM, July 25, 1945.

10. "The Shawmut Mining Co.," *Kane* (PA) *Republican*, October 20, 1945.

CHAPTER 4: THE SIRENS SING

1. Mark's words are cited in the letter from JDD to JM, July 25, 1945, Manuscript Group 52: UMWA District 2, Box 61, Folder 5 and Box 68, Folder 1, Special Collections and University Archives, IUP.

2. JDD to JM, July 25, 1945.

3. Ray Sprigle, "Disease Stalks Company Villages," *Pittsburgh Post-Gazette*, August 17, 1945.

4. "Woman Doctor, Miners Quit in Fight to Clean Up Coal Towns," *Pittsburgh Press*, July 31, 1945.

5. "State Probing Insanitation at Coal Towns," *Pittsburgh Press*, August 1, 1945.

6. Associated Press, "Doctor, Miners Quit in Protest," *Rocky Mount* (NC) *Telegram*, August 1, 1945.

7. Associated Press, "Shawmut Mine Town to Get Real Cleanup," *Daily American* (Somerset, PA), August 2, 1945.

8. United Press, "State Orders 4 Towns in Valley to Boil Water," *Courier-Express* (DuBois, PA), August 2, 1945.

9. United Press, "State Orders 4 Towns in Valley to Boil Water."

10. Elaine Kahn Light, sound recording, National Council of Jewish Women, Pittsburgh Section, June 9, 1992, Tape 1, Side 2.

11. Light, sound recording.

12. "Former Kingston Doctor Will Quit Mining Town," *Wilkes-Barre* (PA) *Record,* August 2, 1945.

13. Elaine Kahn for the Associated Press, "Mine Company Promises Cleanup of 'Intolerable' Sanitary Conditions," *Harrisburg* (PA) *Telegraph*, August 2, 1945.

14. Judy Shepard, "Striking Miners Refuse to Betray 'Dr. Betty,'" *New York Post*, August 2, 1945.

15. Shepard, "Striking Miners Refuse to Betray 'Dr. Betty.'"

16. Kahn, "Mine Company Promises Cleanup of 'Intolerable' Sanitary Conditions."

17. Julia Shawell, "Woman Doctor Leaving; It's Okay with Coal Co.," *Philadelphia Record*, August 2, 1945.

18. Julia Shawell, "Striking Miners Act to Back Woman Doctor's Cleanup Fight; Ask Unemployment Compensation, Won't Work without Her," *Philadelphia Record*, August 3, 1945.

19. Stanley Frank and Paul Sann, "Paper Dolls," *Saturday Evening Post*, May 20, 1944, 93.

20. Editorial, "An Indignant Physician Prescribes for All of Us," *Philadelphia Record*, August 3, 1945.

21. Editorial, "Dr. Betty Does a Job," *Pittsburgh Press*, August 3, 1945.

22. "'Dr. Betty' Blisters State's Failure to Purify Wells," *Pittsburgh Press*, August 3, 1945.

23. "Force Situation Is Unchanged, Survey Is Nearing Completion," *Courier-Express* (DuBois, PA), August 4, 1945.

24. "Doctor Fighting for Miners 'Keeping Faith' with Father," *Pittsburgh Press*, August 5, 1945.

25. "Doctor Fighting for Miners 'Keeping Faith' with Father."

26. "State Wants Mining Town Cleaned Up," *Wilkes-Barre* (PA) *Times Leader*, August 8, 1945.

27. "Former Kingston Doctor Will Quit Mining Town."

28. Hilton Wick, "Doctors Are Funny Folks, Shouts Wick," *Leader-Vindicator* (Bethlehem, PA), August 8, 1945.

29. The account of the community meeting and associated quotes are from "Miners Ask for Showdown on Pure Water," *Pittsburgh Press*, August 10, 1945.

30. "Gavin Finds That Conditions in Mine Town Are Terrible," *News-Herald* (Franklin, PA), August 13, 1945.

31. Sprigle, "Disease Stalks Company Villages."

32. Sprigle, "Disease Stalks Company Villages."

33. United Press, "Force Miners Appeal to Gov. Edward Martin, John L. Lewis to Rectify Sanitary Conditions," *Clearfield* (PA) *Progress*, August 25, 1945.

34. C. M. Enochs, Powers Dixon, and Dennis Burns to John L. Lewis, April 5, 1946, reprinted in ad, *Knoxville* (TN) *News-Sentinel*, May 11, 1946.

35. United Press, "Force Miners Appeal to Gov. Edward Martin."

36. "Strikers Backing 'Dr. Betty' Called Up for Induction," *Pittsburgh Press*, August 13, 1945.

37. "DuBois to Stage Victory Parade Tonight at 7:00," *Courier-Express* (DuBois, PA), August 15, 1945.

38. "V-J Day Frees Miners to Move as Cleanup Is Started in Valley," *Courier-Express* (DuBois, PA), August 15, 1945.

39. Kahn, "Mine Company Promises Cleanup of 'Intolerable' Sanitary Conditions."

40. Chester Potter, "Mining Firm's Debts Pyramid in Record 40-Year Receivership," *Pittsburgh Press*, August 8, 1945.

41. Potter, "Mining Firm's Debts Pyramid in Record 40-Year Receivership."

42. Sprigle, "Disease Stalks Company Villages."

43. "Shawmut Miners Plan Mass Emigration," *Courier-Express* (DuBois, PA), August 18, 1945.

CHAPTER 5: CRACKS AND PATCHES

1. Ray Sprigle, "Disease Stalks Company Villages," *Pittsburgh Post-Gazette*, August 17, 1945.

2. Ray Sprigle, "Company Financing Smells of Slums," *Pittsburgh Post-Gazette*, August 18, 1945.

3. Sprigle, "Company Financing Smells of Slums."

4. Sprigle, "Company Financing Smells of Slums."

5. Ray Sprigle, "Squalid Houses Pay Rich Dividends," *Pittsburgh Post-Gazette*, August 20, 1945.

6. Sprigle, "Squalid Houses Pay Rich Dividends."

7. Sprigle, "Squalid Houses Pay Rich Dividends."

8. "Force Woman Shoots Self, Dies Here," *Courier-Express* (DuBois, PA), August 23, 1945.

9. "Force Miners Call on Lewis for Aid in Sanitation Fight," *Pittsburgh Press*, August 25, 1945.

10. The account of the community meeting comes from an August 24, 1945, letter from Anthony Coccimiglio to John L. Lewis, UMWA President's Office correspondence with districts, Pennsylvania State University Special Collections Library.

11. Ray Sprigle, "Miners Seek to Extend Fight for Sanitation," *Pittsburgh Post-Gazette*, August 25, 1945.

12. John J. Mattes to Anthony Coccimiglio, August 25, 1945, UMWA President's Office correspondence, Pennsylvania State University.

13. John L. Lewis to Edward Lewellen, September 6, 1945, UMWA President's Office correspondence, Pennsylvania State University.

14. "Force Miners to Receive Jobless Compensation," *Pittsburgh Post-Gazette*, August 30, 1945.

15. Elizabeth Gurley Flynn, "Coal Miners in the Headlines," *Daily Worker*, August 13, 1945.

16. Walter Lowenfels, "Dr. 'Betty,'" *Daily Worker*, August 26, 1945.

17. "UMW Won't Aid Health Strike," *New York Post*, August 28, 1945.

18. Elizabeth Gurley Flynn, "Lewis Silent as Miners Drink Sewage," *Daily Worker*, September 9, 1945.

19. "Shawmut to Oppose Idle Compensation," *Courier-Express* (DuBois, PA), September 1, 1945.

20. "Force Miners to Receive Jobless Compensation."

21. "Force Strikers Appeal Case to President," *Pittsburgh Press*, September 6, 1945.

22. "Force Strikers Appeal Case to President."

23. "Force Strikers Appeal Case to President."

24. Chester Potter, "Mining Firm's Debts Pyramid in Record 40-Year Receivership," *Pittsburgh Press*, August 8, 1945.

25. This and subsequent Dickson quotes are in a letter from JDD to JM, September 7, 1945, Manuscript Group 52: UMWA District 2, Box 61, Folder 5 and Box 68, Folder 1, Special Collections and University Archives, IUP.

26. All quotes from the *Baltimore Sun* article from Katherine Scarborough, "Dr. Betty's Own Strike Still Ties Up Mines," *Baltimore Sun*, September 9, 1945.

CHAPTER 6: THE FEDS AND THE GOON

1. William D. Hassett to the U.S. Department of Justice, General File, Harry S. Truman Library, September 6, 1945.

2. George Zielke, "Probe of Mining Town Receivership Ordered," *Pittsburgh Post-Gazette*, September 7, 1945.

3. Howard Ball, *Hugo L. Black: Cold Steel Warrior* (New York: Oxford University Press, 1996), 97.

4. Elizabeth Gurley Flynn, "Lewis Silent as Miners Drink Sewage," *Daily Worker,* September 9, 1945.

5. Ray Sprigle, "U.S. Probes Shawmut Coal Firm," *Pittsburgh Post-Gazette,* September 18, 1945.

6. Editorial, *Philadelphia Record*, September 19, 1945.

7. United Press, "Force Miners Appeal to Gov. Edward Martin, John L. Lewis to Rectify Sanitary Conditions," *Clearfield* (PA) *Progress*, August 25, 1945.

8. Sprigle, "U.S. Probes Shawmut Coal Firm."

9. "Shawmut Co.'s Mounting Debt Probed," *Pittsburgh Press*, September 23, 1945.

10. "Force Strikers Appeal Case to President," *Pittsburgh Press*, September 6, 1945.

11. All letters from RS to CFHA from PS&N Papers, Box 1, Vol. 3 and Box 2, Folder 28, Division of Rare and Manuscript Collections, Cornell University.

12. All remarks from the strike meeting from Ray Sprigle, "Striking Shawmut Miners Smash Back-to-Work Move," *Pittsburgh Post-Gazette*, September 27, 1945.

13. Letter from RS to CFHA, October 2, 1945, PS&N Papers.

14. Bill Davidson, "Dr. Betty," *Salute* 1, no. 1 (April 1946), 47.

15. "No Change in Shawmut Co. Conditions," *Indiana* (PA) *Evening Gazette*, October 11, 1945.

16. "Shawmut Coal Company Ordered to File Receivership Data," *Brockway* (PA) *Record*, October 19, 1945.

17. "Shawmut Coal Company Ordered to File Receivership Data."

18. "This is the U.S.A.," *To Dragma*, October 1945, 14.

19. Gabe Kish and Roy Hudson, "'Force, Pa.' Symbolizes Miners' Fight for Decent Communities," *Sunday Worker*, October 28, 1945.

20. Associated Press, "Referee Upholds Compensation for Force Strikers," *Gazette and Daily* (York, PA), October 31, 1945.

21. "Refereee Upholds Benefits Ruling in Mine Strike," *Harrisburg* (PA) *Telegraph*, October 30, 1945.

22. Ray Sprigle, "If It Isn't Romance, Then What Is It?" *Pittsburgh Post-Gazette*, November 10, 1945.

23. "Shawmut Receiver Removal Sought," *Pittsburgh Press*, November 7, 1945.

24. Letter from RS to CFHA, November 19, 1945, PS&N Papers.

25. Judge Henry Hipple, Opinion, *Commonwealth of Pennsylvania v. F. D. Lambert, David Bell Sr., and Francis Erich*, January sessions, 1946.

CHAPTER 7: MARAUDERS

1. The account of Hayes's eviction is from Bill Davidson, "Dr. Betty," *Salute* 1, no. 1 (April 1946), 47.

2. "Doctor's Office Shut by Mine Executives," *Pittsburgh Post-Gazette*, November 11, 1945.

3. Davidson, "Dr. Betty," 47.

4. Chester Potter, "Dr. Betty Hales Shawmut to Court, Still Aids Miners Without Equipment," *Pittsburgh Press*, November 20, 1945.

5. "Doctor's Office Shut by Mine Executives."

6. Potter, "Dr. Betty Hales Shawmut to Court."

7. Potter, "Dr. Betty Hales Shawmut to Court."

8. Judge Henry Hipple, Opinion, *Commonwealth of Pennsylvania v. F. D. Lambert, David Bell Sr., and Francis Erich*, January sessions, 1946.

9. "Shawmut Coal Officials Trailed by Constable," *Pittsburgh Post-Gazette*, November 20, 1945.

10. "Miners' Resentment Runs High Over Dr. Betty's Eviction," *Pittsburgh Press*, November 20, 1945.

11. For a discussion of images of miners, see Janet Wells Greene, "Cameras in the Coalfields: Photographs as Evidence for Comparative Coalfield History," in *Towards a Comparative History of Coalfield Studies* (Aldershot, Hampshire, UK: Ashgate, 2005), 65–82.

12. Potter, "Dr. Betty Hales Shawmut to Court."

13. This and subsequent Pentz quotes from Chester Potter, "Shawmut Miners Offer Peace Plan," *Pittsburgh Press*, November 21, 1945.

14. "Shawmut Strikers Charge Jobless Pay Shenanigans," *Pittsburgh Press*, November 23, 1945.

15. Associated Press, "Receivership of Dickson Ruins Assets," *Daily American* (Somerset, PA), November 22, 1945.

16. Potter, "Shawmut Miners Offer Peace Plan."

17. "Popular Hollywood Girl Is Instantly Killed by Passing Car," *Courier-Express* (DuBois, PA), November 24, 1945.

CHAPTER 8: FEET TO THE FIRE

1. "An Opened Book," *Business Week*, November 17, 1945, 79.

2. John F. Fitzgerald, letter to the editor, *Pittsburgh Post-Gazette*, November 23, 1945.

3. Ruth MacKay, "White Collar Girl," *Chicago Daily Tribune*, December 18, 1945.

4. "Stagnation and History on the PS&N R.R.," *Investor's Weekly*, December 19, 1945, 22.

5. Associated Press, "Doctor Testifies at Hearing for Area Railroad," *Rochester* (NY) *Democrat and Chronicle*, November 28, 1945.

6. Bill Davidson, "Dr. Betty," *Salute* 1, no. 1 (April 1946), 47.

7. Ray Sprigle, "Shawmut Receiver Removal Will Be Decided Today," *Pittsburgh Post-Gazette*, November 28, 1945.

8. "Dr. Betty in Court Here for Fight on Receivership," *Pittsburgh Press*, November 27, 1945.

9. Sprigle, "Shawmut Receiver Removal Will Be Decided Today."

10. Sprigle, "Shawmut Receiver Removal Will Be Decided Today."

11. Sprigle, "Shawmut Receiver Removal Will Be Decided Today."

12. "Receiver Is Questioned on Purchase," *Wilkes-Barre* (PA) *Times Leader*, November 28, 1945.

13. Sprigle, "Shawmut Receiver Removal Will Be Decided Today."

14. Associated Press, "Dr. 'Betty' Testifies to Shocking Lack of Sanitation in Shawmut Hearing," *Gazette and Daily* (York, PA), November 28, 1945.

15. Rudy Cernkovic for the United Press, "Seek to Oust Shawmut Head," *News-Herald* (Franklin, PA), November 28, 1945.

16. Associated Press, "Cracks in Houses at Force So Big Cats Could Be Thrown Through Them, Bard Is Told," *Wilkes-Barre* (PA) *Record*, November 28, 1945.

17. Associated Press, "Cracks in Houses at Force So Big Cats Could Be Thrown Through Them, Bard Is Told."

18. Associated Press, "Charges Hurled at Receivership in Shawmut Case," *Oil City* (PA) *Derrick*, November 27, 1945.

19. Cernkovic, "Seek to Oust Shawmut Head."

20. Associated Press, "Charges Hurled at Receivership in Shawmut Case."

21. The account of, and quotes from, the Force contingent waiting for the verdict from Davidson, "Dr. Betty."

22. "Shawmut Receiver Ousted by Court," *Pittsburgh Post-Gazette*, November 29, 1945.

23. Daily Feature and Pictorial Page, *Philadelphia Inquirer*, November 29, 1945.

24. "State Medical Society Supports Dr. Betty Hayes," *Pittsburgh Press*, November 29, 1945.

25. "Dr Betty Scores Victory in Railroad Feud," *Business Week*, December 1, 1945, 108.

26. "At Shawmut, Strike to End," *Pittsburgh Press*, December 1, 1945.

27. "Stagnation and History on the PS&N R.R.," 23.

28. Ray Sprigle, "Shawmut Miners, Softened Up, Return to Pits—Now Backs Ache," *Pittsburgh Post-Gazette*, December 11, 1945.

29. "At Shawmut, Strike to End."

30. Editorial, "Not Always Golden," *Daily Press* (St. Marys, PA), November 29, 1945.

31. Editorial, "Not Always Golden."

32. Letter from JDD to JM, September 7, 1945, Manuscript Group 52: UMWA District 2, Box 61, Folder 5 and Box 68, Folder 1, Special Collections and University Archives, IUP.

33. Cernkovic, "Seek to Oust Shawmut Head."

34. United Press, "Five Months' Strike to End, Shawmut Miners Return Monday," *Daily Republican* (Monongahela, PA), December 7, 1945.

35. Letter from RS to CFHA, December 2, 1945, PS&N Papers, Box 1, Vol. 3 and Box 2, Folder 28, Division of Rare and Manuscript Collections, Cornell University.

36. RS to CFHA, December 2, 1945.

37. "New Receiver Angelica Boy," *Evening Tribune* (Hornell, NY), December 19, 1923.

38. Lee Cory, *Stories of the Pittsburg, Shawmut & Northern Railroad* (Angelica, NY: Pittsburgh, Shawmut & Northern Railroad Company Historical Society, 1993), 91–92.

39. "Dr. Betty Cleans Up," *Time*, December 24, 1945, 95.

40. Letter from RS to CFHA, January 23, 1946, PS&N Papers.

41. "Dr. 'Betty' Hayes Speaks on Mining Town at Lions Meet," *News-Herald* (Franklin, PA), January 11, 1946.

42. "It Happened in the USA," *International Stereotypers and Electrotypers Union Journal*, January 1, 1946, 23.

CHAPTER 9: RESCUE TEAM

1. Associated Press, "State Rests in Coal Trial," *Indiana* (PA) *Evening Gazette*, January 17, 1946.

2. Commonwealth's Points for Charge, *Commonwealth of Pennsylvania v. F. D. Lambert, David Bell, Sr., and Francis Erich*, January sessions, no. 33, February 13, 1946.

3. "Shawmut-Hayes Case Reaches Jury Today," *Ridgway* (PA) *Record*, January 16, 1946.

4. Judge Henry Hipple, Opinion, *Commonwealth of Pennsylvania v. F. D. Lambert, David Bell Sr., and Francis Erich*, January sessions, 1946.

5. Associated Press, "Shawmut Case Goes to Jury," *Pittsburgh Sun-Telegraph*, January 16, 1946.

6. "Verdict Is Reached in Shawmut Case," *Ridgway* (PA) *Record*, January 17, 1946.

7. Letter from RS to CFHA, January 23, 1946, PS&N Papers, Box 1, Vol. 3 and Box 2, Folder 28, Division of Rare and Manuscript Collections, Cornell University.

8. Associated Press, "Lease Starts New Chapter on Shawmut Case," *Bradford* (PA) *Era*, February 1, 1946.

9. "Lease-Sales Offer Made for Shawmut," *Pittsburgh Post-Gazette*, January 24, 1946.

10. Letter from RS to CFHA, January 28, 1946, PS&N Papers.

11. Ray Sprigle, "Court Signs Shawmut Mine Lease Order," *Pittsburgh Post-Gazette*, February 1, 1946.

12. Sprigle, "Court Signs Shawmut Mine Lease Order."

13. Resolution Committees of Locals 97 and 6397 to the United Mine Workers of America, January 23, 1946.

14. Resolution Committees of Locals 97 and 6397 to the United Mine Workers of America.

15. Resolution Committees of Locals 97 and 6397 to the United Mine Workers of America.

16. Associated Press, "Freedom Menaced," *Montana Standard* (Butte, MT), February 8, 1946.

17. Ted Allen, "Coal Camps Never Knew Modern Living Conditions," *Sunday Worker,* April 7, 1946.

18. Letter from RS to CFHA, February 21, 1946, PS&N Papers.

19. Associated Press, "Dr. Sherman Quits Industrial Surgery to Write Book," *Pittsburgh Sun-Telegraph*, February 21, 1946.

20. Letter from RS to CFHA, April 1, 1946, PS&N Papers.

21. News item, *Daily Press* (St. Marys, PA), March 14, 1946.

22. Editorial, "Rumors Denied," *Daily Press* (St. Marys, PA), April 4, 1946.

23. Louis Stark, "Lewis and Leader of Mine Operators in Clash at Parley," *New York Times*, March 15, 1946.

24. Associated Press, "Mine Owners, Lewis Reject Safety Offers," *Chicago Daily Tribune*, April 3, 1946.

25. *Congressional Record* S5476, May 23, 1946.

26. *Congressional Record* S5476.

27. Wayne Thomis, "Mine Camp Sunk in Squalor, But Few Try to Rise," *Chicago Tribune*, May 18, 1946.

28. Letter from RS to CFHA, April 1, 1946, PS&N Papers.

29. Editorial, "Is St. Marys Interested in Saving Shawmut Line?" *Daily Press* (St. Marys, PA), April 30, 1946.

CHAPTER 10: REVERBERATIONS

1. Judge Henry Hipple, Opinion, *Commonwealth of Pennsylvania v. F. D. Lambert, David Bell Sr., and Francis Erich*, January sessions, 1946.

2. Hipple, Opinion,

3. Letter from RS to CFHA, May 7, 1946, PS&N Papers, Box 1, Vol. 3 and Box 2, Folder 28, Division of Rare and Manuscript Collections, Cornell University.

4. Editorial, "Concrete Steps Taken," *Daily Press* (St. Marys, PA), May 17, 1946.

5. Letter from RS to CFHA, May 15, 1946, PS&N Papers.

6. Lewis Stark, "Krug Takes Over; Lewis Is Said to Put Decision to Work for U.S. Up to Individuals," *New York Times*, May 22, 1946.

7. United Press, "The Text of the Bituminous Coal Agreement," *New York Times*, May 30, 1946.

8. U.S. Department of the Interior, *A Medical Survey of the Bituminous-Coal Industry: Report of the Coal Mines Administration* (Washington, DC: U.S. Government Printing Office, 1947). This is also referred to as the Boone report.

9. Ray Sprigle, "Company Financing Smells of Slums," *Pittsburgh Post-Gazette,* August 18, 1945.

10. U.S. Department of the Interior, *A Medical Survey of the Bituminous-Coal Industry,* xxiv.

11. "Winning Hearts and Mines: Dr. Joel Boone and the Bituminous Coal Medical Survey of 1947," *The Grog,* Summer 2011, 6.

12. U.S. Department of the Interior, *A Medical Survey of the Bituminous-Coal Industry,* xxiv.

13. "Shawmut Coal Receivers Get More Authority," *Pittsburgh Press,* August 13, 1946.

14. Letter from RS to CFHA, August 23, 1946, PS&N Papers.

15. RS to CFHA, August 23, 1946.

16. Editorial, "To Voice Protest," *Daily Press* (St. Marys, PA), August 23, 1946.

17. "Coal Town's Sanitation Denounced," *Pittsburgh Post-Gazette,* November 7, 1946.

18. United Press, "State's Coal Areas Reported Sanitary," *Pittsburgh Press,* November 8, 1946.

19. U.S. Department of the Interior, *A Medical Survey of the Bituminous-Coal Industry,* 11.

20. U.S. Department of the Interior, *A Medical Survey of the Bituminous-Coal Industry,* 73.

21. U.S. Department of the Interior, *A Medical Survey of the Bituminous-Coal Industry,* 71.

22. Ray Sprigle, "Shawmut Mining Towns Rise Out of Slough with Prospects of New Comfort by Spring," *Pittsburgh Post-Gazette,* December 26, 1946.

23. "In a Paragraph," *Kane* (PA) *Republican,* November 22, 1946.

24. Sprigle, "Shawmut Mining Towns Rise Out of Slough."

25. Sprigle, "Shawmut Mining Towns Rise Out of Slough."

26. Sprigle, "Shawmut Mining Towns Rise Out of Slough."

27. "Shawmut Line Abandonment Recommended," *Pittsburgh Post-Gazette,* November 21, 1946.

28. "Three Elk County Towns Awakened When 'Dr. Betty' Begins Crusade," *Grit,* February 2, 1947, 14.

CHAPTER 11: FAREWELL TO THE VALLEY

1. Editorial, "Ray of Hope," *Daily Press* (St. Marys, PA), February 7, 1947.

2. Editorial, "Monday, March 3," *Daily Press* (St. Marys, PA), March 1, 1947.

3. "Shawmut Company Sold for 1½ Millions," *Pittsburgh Press,* March 3, 1947.

4. Editorial, "A Dynasty Ends," *Daily Press* (St. Marys, PA), March 4, 1947.

5. Editorial, "A Railroad Dies," *Daily Press* (St. Marys, PA), March 4, 1947.

6. "PS&N Sale Ends Oldest Receivership," *Railway Age* 122, no. 13 (March 29, 1947), 654–55.

7. Editorial, "End of a Receivership," *Pittsburgh Press*, March 6, 1947.

8. Elizabeth Gurley Flynn, "Calling All Women," *The Worker* (supplement to the *Daily Worker*), March 9, 1947.

9. Flynn, "Calling All Women."

10. "Force Physician Kiwanis Speaker," *Kane* (PA) *Republican*, January 21, 1947.

11. U.S. Department of the Interior, *A Medical Survey of the Bituminous-Coal Industry: Report of the Coal Mines Administration* (Washington, DC: U.S. Government Printing Office, 1947), 60.

12. Associated Press, "'Dr. Betty' Quitting Miners' Valley," *Pittsburgh Sun-Telegraph*, June 9, 1947; "Miners' Picnic Honors Dr. Betty," *Pittsburgh Press*, June 9, 1947.

13. Ray Sprigle, "Dr. Betty Says Goodbye to Bennett's Valley," *Pittsburgh Post-Gazette*, June 9, 1947.

14. "Main Street in Coaltown USA," *Daily Worker*, June 29, 1947.

15. Associated Press, "'Dr. Betty' Quitting Miners' Valley."

EPILOGUE

1. Nancy Huffman, telephone interview with the author, June 27, 2019.

2. "Bennett's Valley Fighting for Better Phones," *Courier-Express* (DuBois, PA), June 29, 1947.

3. "Shawmut Coal Co. Purchases Big Bituminous Coal Marketing Firm," *Progress* (Clearfield, PA), May 8, 1951.

4. Larry Voris, telephone interview with the author, January 25, 2019.

5. "Eating the Pan," *Indianapolis News*, August 18, 1969.

6. "Slipping Away: Erosion on the Estuarine Coast," *University of North Carolina Sea Grant College Newsletter*, November 1976, 5.

7. Larry Voris interview, January 25, 2019.

BIBLIOGRAPHY

Cory, Lee. *Stories of the Pittsburg, Shawmut & Northern Railroad.* Angelica, NY: Pittsburg, Shawmut & Northern Railroad Company Historical Society, 1993.

Davidson, Bill. "Dr. Betty." *Salute* 1, no. 1 (April 1946), 6–8 and 46–48.

Greene, Janet Wells. "Cameras in the Coalfields: Photographs as Evidence for Comparative Coalfield History." Chapter 4 in *Towards a Comparative History of Coalfield Societies.* Aldershot, Hampshire, UK: Ashgate, 2005.

"PS&N Sale Ends Oldest Receivership," *Railway Age* 122, no. 13 (March 29, 1947), 654–55.

Sprigle, Ray. "Plague Spots" series. *Pittsburgh Post-Gazette*, August 17, 18, and 20, 1945.

U.S. Department of the Interior. *A Medical Survey of the Bituminous-Coal Industry: Report of the Coal Mines Administration.* Washington, DC: U.S. Government Printing Office, 1947.

Walsh, Mary Roth. *"Doctors Wanted: No Women Need Apply": Sexual Barriers in the Medical Profession, 1835–1975.* New Haven, CT: Yale University Press, 1977.

FREQUENTLY CITED PERIODICALS

Courier-Express (DuBois, PA)
Daily Press (St. Marys, PA)
Daily Worker
Philadelphia Record
Pittsburgh Post-Gazette
Pittsburgh Press

ACKNOWLEDGMENTS

First, I would like to thank Dave Wulderk for his generosity and encouragement. Through his talks and research, Dave has kept the memory of Dr. Betty Hayes alive in the area around Force. I'm in awe of his work and grateful for his help. I also had the indispensable aid of archivists and librarians at the Special Collections and University Archives at Indiana University of Pennsylvania, the Division of Rare and Manuscript Collections at Cornell University, the Special Collections Library at Penn State, the Historical Society of Pennsylvania, the Heinz History Center, the New York Academy of Medicine, and my beloved New York Public Library. The Elk County Historical Society and the St. Marys Public Library kindly let me use their digital newspaper archives. I'm indebted to Dr. Hayes's niece, Nancy Huffman, and stepson, Larry Voris, for sharing their memories of her. Perry Winkler, a nephew of strike leader Norman Winkler, gave me a glimpse into the past, and Richard Liskov answered some pressing questions. I thank my editor, Jake Bonar, and my agent, Amanda Jain, for their belief in this project. Finally, special thanks to Michael, Jonah, Phyllis, and Paul for all their egging-on and putting-up-with.